Brian, Balance

D1132093

An Undetected Acid-Alkaline Imbalance

WARNING

Acid and Excess Proteins Are Slowly Killing You And Severely Hurting Your Children!

The First Book in North America that Details An Undetected Acid-Alkaline Imbalance and Its Relationship to the Lymphatic System and the Disease Process

John Ossipinsky LMT, CST-D, LLCC
Diplomate Certified CranioSacral Therapist
Certified Lymphedema Therapist

An Undetected Acid-Alkaline Imbalance

By John Ossipinsky, LMT, CST-D, LLCC

Published by: Vision Publishing, LLC
P.O. Box 2122
Wickenburg, AZ 85358

Copyright © 2006, 2009 by John Ossipinsky

All rights reserved. No part of this book may be reproduced or transmitted in any form or by means, electronic or mechanical, including but not limited to, photocopying, recording, slides, electronic mail, internet, or by any information or storage system without written permission from the author, except for the inclusion of brief quotations in a review.

An Undetected Acid-Alkaline Imbalance

Library of Congress Control Number: 2008937264

ISBN Print Edition: 978-0-9774917-2-8

First Printing 2006
Second Printing 2009, revised

1. Health. 2. Nutrition. 3. Self-Help.

Printed in the United States of America

Superficial Lymph Circulation of the Torso

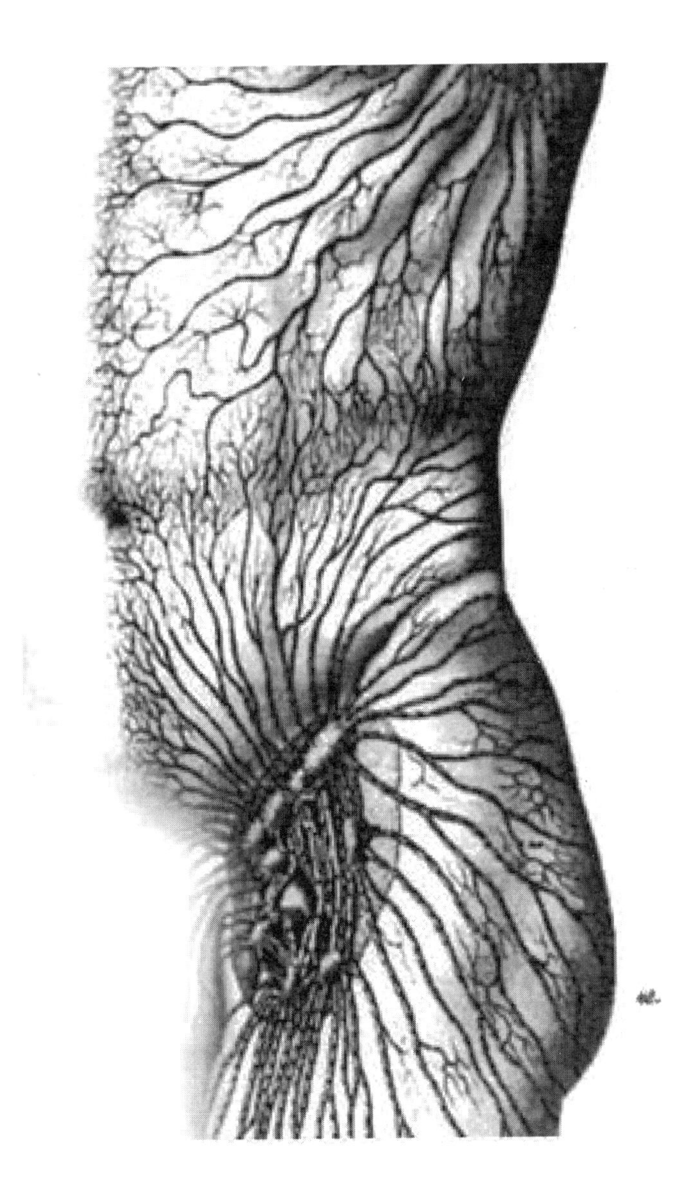

From *Silent Waves* by Dr. Chikly, used with permission

An Undetected Acid-Alkaline Imbalance

DISCLAIMER

The material contained in this book is for information only and is not meant to be used for self-diagnosis or as a substitute for consultation with a health care provider. The information is not intended to replace medical advice offered by physicians. If you have any questions about any disease described within this book, consult a health care provider.

The author, editors, or publishers are not responsible for any errors or omissions or for the results obtained from the use of such material. They make no representations or warranties with respect to any treatment, action, or application of nutritional supplements, medication or preparation by any person following the information offered or provided within this book and will not be liable for any direct, indirect, consequential, special, exemplary, or other damages arising there from. You agree to hold harmless and indemnify the authors, editors, or publishers, against any liability for any claims and expenses, including reasonable attorney's fees, relating to any violation of the terms of this agreement or arising out of any materials submitted by you.

Readers are encouraged to confirm the information contained herein with other sources and carefully review the accuracy of the information with their professional health care provider. Before changing your dietary and exercise habits consult with a professional health care provider. Never stop any medication without consulting your health care provider.

An Undetected Acid-Alkaline Imbalance

DEDICATION

My loving wife Eileen, when we married we became partners in love and in life. I know our life has always been a roller coaster, with many high-speed turns and a few low bumps. Thank you for tightening your seat belt, taking a deep breath and always being by my side. Our deep love has always been our strength. Most of all, thank you, for your patience and tireless efforts in helping me bring this important information to life. Without you it would have been an "Impossible Dream."

My wise children, Falin and Colin, you always put a smile on my lips and in my heart. You are my inspiration in life and for this book. As a parent I only want good things for you, especially good health. I hope this book helps guide you in the many decisions ahead in your life. With the right information, you can make the right choices. Thank you for showing me the importance of this undetected acid-alkaline imbalance. Your endless love and support, especially all your hugs and kisses have made each day a special one.

My parents, Vincenza and John J., thank you, for always loving and supporting me and for opening my eyes to so many different experiences in life. Thank you for showing me how a committed, loving relationship takes effort and communication to last.

Those who have graciously helped me with this endeavor, I thank you, for all your hard work and support.

My family, friends, patients and the public if you gain one piece of information from this book that may improve your or your family's quality of life and future, my task would be complete.

ACKNOWLEDGEMENTS

This book would not have been possible if my eyes were not first opened to the craniosacral, visceral (organs) and lymphatic systems of the body. For this I have to thank doctors John Upledger, D.O., Jean-Pierre Barral, D.O., and Bruno Chikly, M.D., D.O. (hon). These doctors selflessly decided to show others their work, so that many more people can be helped by their gentle, but life altering therapies. My thanks must be extended to the doctor's many talented instructors and staff at the Upledger Institute, for their dedication in helping to educate others.

After learning about the many systems of the body in detail for over a decade, I met two other doctors whose information allowed me to see the problem of tissue acidosis and the idea of protein proliferation in the body. The term acid-alkaline balance was out of my vocabulary until John Desgrey, N.D. explained the phenomenon to me. I was then fortunate to hear William Wong, N.D., explain how surgery and trauma cause protein proliferation in the body. As information from the doctors came together with later data from my studies, I realized our nation, and the world, is dealing with the negative affects of An Undetected Acid-Alkaline Imbalance.

An Undetected Acid-Alkaline Imbalance

WARNING

Acid and Excess Proteins
Are Slowly Killing You
And Severely
Hurting Your Children!

TABLE OF CONTENTS

INTRODUCTION

There is a Problem!

You may be questioning whether the title of this book, An Undetected Acid-Alkaline Imbalance, is true. Is there a major health problem, an imbalance, that we are unaware of? Yes, there is a major problem. Many of you are tired, overweight, sick and don't even know the real cause. In writing this book I hope to show you how an undetected acid-alkaline imbalance is constricting your lymphatic system which leads to toxicity in your internal body. This imbalance is slowing the ability of your lymphatic system to clean your tissues and organs. When you think of the lymphatic system, picture it as a sewage treatment plant for your body. When the lymphatic system is not able to work efficiently, fluid, acidic cellular waste, excess proteins such as fibrin and parts of dead cells and toxins can build in your tissues. As these toxins build, you can become tired, tight and sick. If I stopped cleaning my fish tank, over time the fluid environment will become dirty, toxic and negatively affect the health of the fish. Let me explain this in more detail.

When I was a young boy we had a fish tank with many different fish. The fish were always getting "ich", their eyes would bulge out and their scales would start falling off, many of them died. We were always going to the local pet store for "ich" medication for the fish. The fish would get well for a while and then become ill again. The problem is the fish didn't have a specific disease they just became toxic and sick from swimming in their own urine and feces. You see we didn't clean the filter as often as we should have.

That same scenario is happening in your body today. Your body is the fish tank, your living cells are the fish and your lymphatic system and organs are the filter. You aren't sick, your internal body is toxic and you need to have your filters cleaned. Instead we run to the pharmacy for medication that only deals with the "Symptom" not the "Root Problem of Toxicity." Activating the lymphatic system cleans your filters (skin, organs and lymphatic nodes) allowing for enhanced circulation, detoxification and vibrant health. When you are overly acidic, your inner fluids become toxic and damaging to your cells creating disease. As you become toxic and acidic from the air you breathe medications, pollution, environmental toxins, high acid diets, lack of exercise, excess stress and constant dehydration your lymphatic system and other vessels in the body can become constricted. This leads to limited circulation of blood, oxygen and nutrients through your tissues and organs. Over time this allows a buildup of toxic acidic waste, proteins and environmental toxins to become trapped in and around your cells in your body.

A congested area can become out of balance, extremely toxic and over time may lead to cellular damage and disease in the tissues, i.e., cancer, heart disease, candida, lupus, fibromyalgia, chronic fatigue and multiple sclerosis to name only a few. The idea that you are out balance and filling with your own cellular waste and excess proteins is so important to understand, that the theme will be repeated many times throughout the book.

We Live and Die at the Cellular Level

When you are not feeling well you take your temperature and blood pressure. What you should be checking is the pH, or acid-alkaline level of your body, especially your tissues. It is a very easy test that you can do at home in a matter of minutes with pH test strips. Your health depends on the health of your cells, which group together to become tissue and everything within your body, i.e., skin, muscle, bones, organs and central nervous system.

Many experts agree that "We Live and Die at the Cellular Level." Toxins and excess proteins in your body, many of which we produce through regular cellular metabolism, are creating a toxic, unhealthy internal cellular environment. This toxicity is making your cells, and ultimately your whole being, ill. More unbelievable is that this simple imbalance that is negatively affecting all of us in some way is not used in the idea of disease or how to attain health.

Before September 2003 I had never heard of an acidic pH. I then met naturopathic physician John Desgrey, coauthor of the book "Beyond Pritikin". Dr. Desgrey had come into my office for help in recuperating from an illness. Dr. Desgrey was very interesting to speak with about health. He explained how in the 1970's, Naturopathic doctor's studied food and were finding out that if you ate the right foods your internal body became more in balance. During one of our sessions he told me that my six years of being nauseous, and my lifelong stomach and weight problems, were due to me being out of balance and toxic. That meeting opened my eyes. Dr. Desgrey told me about a pH test that would tell me if I was acidic in a matter of seconds. When I tested myself I was severely acidic at 5.0 on the pH scale. When I tested my wife and two young children, they were also severely acidic. This shocked and terrified me. As a parent I am responsible for the health of my children, yet I wasn't aware that many of their small health problems like hyperactivity, eczema, allergies, earaches or constipation were caused by over acidity and toxicity in their bodies. Worse yet, I was unknowingly promoting this acid imbalance in my children with excessive amounts of acid foods, like processed white flour and drinks like sodas. Many of the foods I thought were healthy were actually making my children more toxic and creating many of their health problems.

A Simple Imbalance

While researching acid-alkaline balance, I found many books written on the subject and an enormous amount of information on the Internet. One theme runs true in most of these books and websites, they state that illness and disease start when the body becomes overly acidic and out of balance. Once you understand the basic science of how this acid imbalance is negatively affecting your lymphatic system, an emerging science, you will agree with the experts and see that excess acid is not healthy for you. You will become outraged as you learn how not understanding this emerging science about the basic functioning of your body has led to a simple imbalance that is making you overly acidic, toxic and slowing killing you.

As this undetected imbalance constricts the lymphatic system and tissues it creates congestion of fluid, acidic waste and protein around your cells. Because the lymphatic system is connected to most systems of the body this congestion can negatively impact every part of your body. This information about acid-alkaline balance and the lymphatic system has been accessible for decades yet we know little about it. Because of this catastrophic oversight, people close to you are becoming sick and dying needlessly. When you learn how to make better choices to reduce acid in your life and to improve your circulation through lymphatic activation you will regain your health.

Some examples of the simple steps in this book are eating a greener diet, using nutritional supplements, exercising, drinking mineralized water, deep breathing, good posture, stress reduction, and self-lymphatic activation to help move your lymph and blood through your tissues. I hope to give you the right information that will empower you to change your life, if you give it a chance.

You will see that diet changes alone are not enough to make you truly healthy. The real missing key to improving your health is lymphatic activation to improve circulation. This can be accomplished through many avenues; some ways that you will learn about in the book are massage therapy, CranioSacral

Therapy, Lymph Drainage Therapy or Lymphatic Cellular Detox Massage self-lymphatic activation. Manually increasing circulation through your tissues and organs to improve detoxification, the removal of waste and toxins, in your body is essential for you to have a healthy and happy life.

Toxins are Everywhere

Environmental toxins really are all around you. In recent studies, perchlorate, a by product of jet fuel is being found in all mothers' breast milk in 36 samples tested across 18 states. The same study found perchlorate in 47 of 48 samples of cow's milk collected from 11 states. This is a problem because perchlorate can cause mental retardation in infants and slow metabolism in adults, among other things. As jet fuel burns, or is released to evaporate into the atmosphere before a plane lands, it eventually becomes part of the air you breathe, your food and water supply. In other studies they are finding dangerous super-toxins like dioxin, a by-product of the manufacturing or burning of polyvinyl chloride (PVC).

Over the past four decades, almost everything being manufactured is made of plastic or contains PVC's. Common PVC products are all around you in car seat covers, clothing, plastic bottles, plastic garbage bags, pen cases, television and computer cases, vinyl siding, the plumbing in your home, even wallpaper. This is a serious problem! Over the past two decades efforts have been made to stop dumping garbage into our oceans, instead many areas have turned to mass-burn incinerators. Much of our waste contains materials made with PVC's. When we burn it, dioxin goes out into our atmosphere and travels for miles to fall to the ground, the ocean, a stream or park or street where your child is playing. When the toxin falls on crops that are later eaten by chickens, cows, steers and pigs, it becomes part of your food chain. These toxins will never go away. To have health you need to learn to detox now, and often, to increase your lymphatic system to help remove damaging toxins like perchlorate, dioxin and other poisons such as lead, mercury or cellular waste from your body.

A Better View of the Working Body

I have always had an interest in the body and health. After retiring from the NYC Fire Department I moved to Arizona and was drawn to massage therapy school. Over the next decade I studied the work of three world renowned doctors. Their views of the body and health are very different from traditional medical doctors. These doctors see the body as a whole, where your symptom of shoulder pain may be the result of limited circulation and congestion in the body. These doctors developed hands-on approaches to find and gently release restrictions in the tissues of the body. Releasing these restricted and tight areas allows for improved circulation through your tissues and organs. This improves the fluid environment around your cells and allows the body's own healing mechanisms to begin working. The key is increased circulation.

In 1995 I started learning the work of John Upledger, D.O., developer of CranioSacral Therapy (CST). Dr. Upledger has published many books on this subject, his first book, CranioSacral Therapy was published in 1983. This powerful therapy uses gentle pressure (the weight of a nickel) to release restrictions in the body, especially in the meninges, membranes that surround the brain and spinal cord. When restrictions are released, blood circulation and the ability to heal are enhanced. In CranioSacral Therapy we learn to find and release restricted areas by monitoring tissue tension, energy cysts and the craniosacral rhythm. All are ways to monitor tissue mobility in the body.

I then learned the work of Jean-Pierre Barral, M.D., D.O., who developed Visceral Manipulation. Beginning in 1983 Dr. Barral published his first book of a series on Visceral Manipulation. Your viscera are your organs. This therapy is based on the philosophy that all body systems are inter-related, and concentrates on enhancing mobility and circulation in and around the organs to stop pain and improve health. With Visceral Manipulation you learn to monitor the mobility of the organs and their attachments to the body in order to find and release restrictions in the soft tissues.

In 1996 I began learning the work of Bruno Chikly, M.D., D.O. (hon) who developed Lymph Drainage Therapy (LDT), (Drainage is pronounced like massage). In 2001, Dr. Chikly authored the first comprehensive book on the lymphatic system in North America called *Silent Waves, Theory and Practice of Lymph Drainage Therapy.* This extremely gentle therapy gets to the heart of most of your health problems, which is compromised circulation through the tissues and organs, including your brain. LDT manually enhances your lymph flow, increasing the circulation of lymph and blood around and in your cells. This allows toxic acidic waste and proteins to move into the lymph vessels allowing fresh blood that is full of oxygen and nutrition to move deeper through the tissues and into the cells.

Monitoring Lymph Flow

In Lymph Drainage Therapy we learn to monitor the superficial and deep lymph flow anywhere in the body. Lymph drainage therapists use their hands to map the lymph flow in the tissues, organs or bone. They find congestion and then gently open and enhance the flow of the lymph and blood through the congested tissue.

Lymph Drainage Therapy is very effective at removing acidic waste, toxins and excess proteins from your body. Lymphatic activation increases circulation around your cells, improving your overall health.

A Gentle "Lymphatic Cellular Detox Massage"

As a Licensed Massage Therapist, I have taken many extra steps to become Certified in CranioSacral Therapy and Certified in Lymphedema Therapy. For over ten years my wife owned The Center for Natural Therapy, Inc., a Family Medical Massage and Wellness Center in Glendale, Arizona. At the wellness center we specialized in pain relief, stress relief and detoxification therapies. We used massage, CranioSacral Therapy, Lymph Drainage Therapy and a combination of different soft tissue techniques to relieve pain and improve health, focusing on improving circulation through the soft tissues of the body. In 2008 we closed the center and opened the Lymphatic Wellness Center in Wickenburg, Arizona.

After many years of studying and working with the body, I learned about the well-documented acid-alkaline balance theory. My subsequent studies on this acidic and toxic internal environment, and attempts to find the most effective way to detoxify acidic waste and proteins from the body, led to the development of "Lymphatic Cellular Detox Massage." It is a particular combination of techniques that enhance circulation in the lymphatic, craniosacral and visceral (organ) systems of the body. During a series of lymphatic activation sessions consisting of six sessions over a few weeks, patients release large amounts of acidic waste and proteins. In the past few years we have helped hundreds of individuals go through manual detoxification using the same basic soft tissue techniques to increase circulation.

When patients receive a series of Lymphatic Cellular Detox Massages they quickly experience positive changes. Manual detoxification improves the fluid circulation around the cells. When your cells are healthy overall you feel better, more "alive" and your health problems improve. I have witnessed this again and again and am confident that an undetected tissue acidosis and its negative affect on the lymphatic system is hurting most of us in some way.

Lymphatic Cellular Detox Massage enhances lymph flow and blood circulation to help detoxify acidic waste, toxins and proteins from the body, improving the cells environment and how you feel. Increased circulation changes your cellular environment from a hostile and overly acidic environment to a healthier more alkaline environment.

Since learning about and further researching acid's effect on the body, I have learned that being overly acidic or too alkaline negatively affects your lymphatic system by constricting your tissues. When lymph flow is slowed, blood circulation through your tissues is impeded, creating pockets of acidic fluid and excess proteins. This makes your tissues and organs tight, congested and limits their proper function, as in polycystic kidney disease (PKD), where clear fluid filled cysts congest and impair the kidney.

Prior to learning about an acidic pH, I had been studying and working with the lymphatic and craniosacral systems for eight years. At that time I started asking myself these questions: Why is everyone's lymphatic system not flowing as well as it should? I now know that the reason is an overly acidic internal environment.

A Plethora of Diseases Could Occur

In 1991 Theodore A. Baroody, N.D., D.C., Ph.D. authored Alkalize or Die. He writes; "Lymph fluid flows best in an alkaline medium. When the body is overly acidic it slows, creating one of the most chronic, life threatening situations… the plethora of diseases that occur because of hindered lymph flow and increased tissue acid storage are astounding." He also writes, "Therefore in my opinion, acid wastes literally attack the joints, tissues, muscles, organs and glands causing minor to major dysfunction. If they attack the joints, you might develop arthritis. If they attack the muscles, you could possibly end up with myofibrosis (aching muscles). If they attack the organs and glands, a myriad of illnesses could occur."

After studying and working with the lymphatic system for many years, I understand its critical roles in maintaining health. When I read; "Lymph fluid flows best in an alkaline medium. When the body is overly acidic it slows," I immediately understood the severity of this undetected tissue acidosis. If you are overly acidic your lymphatic system is not functioning optimally, you can fill with fluid, acid waste, proteins, cholesterol, hormones and toxins, which will limit your health.

Lymphatic System is an Emerging Science

When I decided to research acid and the lymphatic system in the Merck Manual, a physician's reference, I was shocked to find the lymphatic system is only mentioned a few times as in immunology and when it is diseased as in lymphoma. The lymphatic system is an emerging science; it has vital documented roles in infection, inflammation, edema and in maintaining the health of your tissues that make up your body. In many places in the Merck Manual they indicate they don't know the cause of many of our diseases. The missing information about overly acidic tissues, or more technically tissue acidosis, and its negative affect on the lymphatic system is why we can't see where many of our diseases start.

Please don't take my word that the lymphatic system is ignored in the understanding of disease. Many of you have heard of Dr. Mehmet Oz, renowned cardiac surgeon, author "Healing from the Heart", frequent guest on the Oprah Show, and his book and show on the Discovery Channel called, "You: The Owners Manual." In 2001 Dr. Chikly asked Dr. Oz to write a few words for the back of his book, Silent Waves. Here is what Dr. Oz wrote: "Lymphatics are the next frontier in human disease. Long ignored because of their subtlety and complexity, the mysteries of our cellular "waste disposal" system have been comprehensively deciphered by Bruno Chikly." This is by no means anything against Dr. Oz; I am just trying to make the point that a well respected Dr., an expert in his field is saying that the lymphatic system is ignored in our idea of disease. I respect and like Dr. Oz and many have learned about the body and benefitted by watching his shows or reading his books.

This undetected tissue acidosis and emerging information about the lymphatic system is not a small oversight. It is earth shaking and the reason why so many of you are tight, sick, diabetic, overweight, depressed and dying. It plays a very large role in childhood diseases and in the epidemic of autism spectrum disorders. In desperation I decided to do whatever was needed to educate others about tissue acidosis, its negative affect on the lymphatic system and how to use this new information to improve your health.

Surgeon General's Responsibility

On the advice of two NIH doctors I collected data from over 100 individuals who fasted and then self tested their saliva pH. Over 90% were acidic (unhealthy) and over 40% of them were severely acidic. The data I collected shows there is a major problem. The results were so clear to me that I spent years trying to contact my local Mayor, Governor, Senator, Congressmen, two local Arizona medical schools (an osteopathic college and a naturopathic college), NIH doctors, The Surgeon General and the President.

After months of calls I made contact with a senior medical advisor in the Surgeon General's office. I sent him a letter with my concerns about our nation having an undetected tissue acidosis. When I spoke with the advisor he was hesitant, but after I persisted he agreed to look at research on the problem if I sent it. Six months later after completing a study of over 100 individuals who self tested their saliva pH, I sent him the results.

The study, which I will discuss in Chapter Three, definitely showed that there could be a problem and that further studies should be done. During our next phone call the advisor asked me "How do you cure this acidosis?" I told him education about eating a greener diet, alkalinizing supplements, improved circulation and stress reduction. When I stopped speaking the advisor joked, "Too bad it isn't a drug, you would be a rich man."

When I spoke with the advisor for the last time a few months later, I offered to come to Washington and do a small test of 1000 federal workers who would volunteer to be tested. He said he couldn't do that and there was nothing further he could do about the matter. He hesitantly suggested I try and get in a study, which may take years. He referred me to a website for another NIH office in order to try to enter a study but they never returned my call or e-mails.

Handbook for Health

Even though I am not a doctor or professional researcher, I am writing this book as a lymphatic therapist who is well educated on the lymphatic system and its role in maintaining the body. Understanding the importance of the lymphatic system, there is no doubt in my mind that there is a severe undetected tissue acidosis within our nation and the world. I am also writing this book as a concerned father and concerned citizen. I want my children, family, friends and others to have a handbook for health that is based on science, not hype.

There is more than enough evidence that proves there is a problem. Action needs to be taken by you for your family's health, and by our government for the health of our great nation. There is no need to panic, if you or your child is sick you need to understand the principles in this book about balancing your life, start by consulting with your health care provider and begin to make small changes in your diet and lifestyle.

The main point that needs to be emphasized is that no matter who you are, no matter how healthy you think you are, you need to self-test your and your family's saliva and urine pH levels and understand the impact it has on your health!

Balance in All You Do

You continually hear that balance in your life is important to achieve happiness. That balance is always teetering, moving between your family, spirituality, work and play. When you concentrate more on one aspect than another, your life becomes out of balance. It happens to most of us when we spend too much time on one aspect of life, the other aspects get short changed. It can be watching sports, computer games, exercising, shopping on the Internet, sex, drugs, alcohol or work. When you are too far to one extreme an imbalance occurs.

This imbalance happens in your personal life and it even happens here on earth. When we put too many toxic chemicals in the air, there is an imbalance that leads to acid rain that is damaging many of our forests and lakes. The one place where balance is needed most is within your internal body. In this book you will learn how a toxic tissue acidosis is slowly filling you with fluid, acidic waste, proteins and toxins. More importantly you will become empowered for life by learning about your lymphatic system and how simple tips regarding lifestyle like diet, exercise, stress reduction and lymphatic activation will help increase your circulation, regain your internal balance and give you back your health and life.

CHAPTER ONE

Acid: It's More Than a Stomach Problem

Take this very seriously. Acid is slowly killing you! Do you know anybody who has stomach problems, constipation, IBS (Irritable Bowel Syndrome), too much stomach acid, bloating or gastro esophageal reflux disease (GERD)? We have been watching commercials for acid indigestion for over 50 years with Alka-Seltzer, Brioschi, Mylanta, Bromoseltzer, Tums and Rolaids. How do you spell relief? Now we see Prevacid, Prilosec and Nexium to name only a few. Acid related stomach problems affect millions worldwide. They are overly acidic due to limited circulation which creates congestion and toxicity in their body. One example is an individual who may have a very thin body, but has a large bloated abdomen that protrudes out in front of them. This is severe acidity and congestion. Your body's chemical makeup changes to acid when you become congested and toxic. If you have acid related health problems you are suffering from excess acidic waste in your tissues called tissue acidosis.

Worldwide yearly sales of antacids have topped 16 billion dollars. We are so accustomed, or desensitized, to people having acid and stomach problems that we see the acid as an inconvenience to our digestive system instead of acid that is attacking our tissues and cells which is slowly killing us. According to doctors I have spoken with swelling is a severe problem affecting many of their patients. This over acidity is constricting the lymphatic system which is causing fluid congestion throughout the body causing swelling. Over acidity allows excess fluid, acidic waste and proteins to build in your tissues damaging cells and leading to disease. This over acidity negatively affects more than your digestion. Many of today's top health problems are caused by over acidity. Some of these are pain, stress, headaches, migraines, ADD, IBS, constipation, loose bowels, indigestion, hemorrhoids, allergies, eczema, rashes, sinus problems, inability to think clearly and red, dry, irritated eyes.

If you have been watching the television lately, you have seen the exponential increase in commercials for prescribed drugs to treat the above problems. Millions of individuals are trying to find relief from their undetected acid related health problems. Without completely understanding how the body actually works with regards to tissue acidosis and its affect on the lymphatic system, the pharmaceutical companies are trying to fix every symptom you have that is actually caused by over acidity. Understanding this, most medications are only band-aids that do not get to the "Root Cause" of your health problems which is tissue acidosis and a malfunctioning lymphatic system. Most of your health problems will go away once you learn to utilize the information in this book to activate your lymph flow and become more in balance.

Look Around You

We don't see this undetected tissue acidosis, even though it is affecting every one of us in some way. Look around you. Do you notice any skin problems such as acne, beauty marks, faded brown or black patches and skin growths? Some specialists make a living freezing or cutting growths off our bodies.

Do you see people who are tight or who have neck and back pain, sciatica, or swelling? How about headaches, migraines or sinus problems? Do you think these problems are normal? They are all signs of tissue acidosis and a malfunctioning lymphatic system that cannot keep up with the buildup of toxic cellular waste in the body. Once you understand this undetected disease called tissue acidosis you will say, "How Did We Miss This Basic Science?"

Two Missing Keys to Your Health

We have been very aware of acid and how it can bring on indigestion or gastric reflux disease. Now it is time to learn how two missed keys to your health are making you toxic and negatively affecting your circulation and health.

The first missing key is an undetected overly acidic and toxic internal body, called tissue acidosis. Even though many people will have signs of this acidosis (i.e. gas, heartburn, bloating, muscle tightness, headaches, depression, constipation, recurring infections, acne, eczema, insomnia or lack of energy) they don't realize they are toxic and are being severely hurt. There are people who may look as though they are very healthy and have no outward visible signs of over acidity. Unfortunately, the acid can be silently damaging the cells that make up their tissues, blood, skin, bones and organs.

The second missing key is the overlooked roles of the lymphatic system, an emerging science. This toxic tissue acidosis has a profound negative affect on the lymphatic system. The lymphatic system is made up of vessels and nodes that are responsible for maintaining the health of your cells and tissues. It has a strong connection to every system in the body; especially the craniosacral system (membranes that surround the brain and spinal cord) that supports and helps maintain the brain.

Even though the lymphatic system and craniosacral system are critical components to your well-being, there is little mention of them in the idea of disease. By missing this undetected tissue acidosis and its negative affect on the physical systems of the body you are blind to the toxicity in your tissues. These missed critical keys to your health are major contributing factors as to why most of you are not as healthy as you should be.

When you are overly acidic your sewage treatment plant for the body is slowed, limiting circulation and the lymphatic system's ability to clean the tissues and organs. This creates fluid congestion in your body, making you toxic. Acid-alkaline balance is well documented in more than eight books over the past few decades, yet the information is not used in the understanding of disease or understood by the general public.

The pH Scale

A pH scale is utilized to determine whether a solution is either acid or alkaline. The initials "pH" stands for "Potential of Hydrogen". pH is a measurement of the concentration of hydrogen ions in a given solution. Because of its mathematical formulation, low pH values (acid) are associated with solutions with high concentrations of hydrogen ions, while high pH values (alkaline) are associated with solutions with low concentrations of hydrogen ions. The typical pH scale ranges from 0 to 14, 0 is a strong acid and has a higher concentration of hydrogen ions - 7 is neutral - 14 is a strong base or alkali and has a lesser concentration of hydrogen ions. The pH scale can go below 0 and above 14.

A difference of one pH unit represents a tenfold, or ten times change. For example, the acidity of a sample with a pH of 6 is ten times more acid than that of a sample with a pH of 7. A difference of 2 units, from 7 to 5, would mean that the acidity is one hundred times greater than it should be.

All current information says that your saliva and urine pH should be between 6.5 and 7.5. The fluid that secretes out of the salivary glands into the saliva is more acidic and becomes less acidic as it mixes with the fluids of the mouth. In my saliva pH study, over 90% of the individuals tested were acidic and over 43% tested were severely acidic (below 5.5 on the pH scale). This is severe acidosis and very damaging to your body.

How Do You Become Acidic?

I want to be very clear; a serious problem does exist. If you eat pasta, chocolate, beef, chicken, fish, bread, eggs or rice and drink coffee, tea, soda, beer or wine, you may be overly acidic. These foods are very acid forming in your body. Unfortunately for most of you, this is your daily diet. You wake up in the morning and start your day with acid in the form of a few cups of coffee or tea, processed orange juice, toast, eggs and bacon. Lunch and dinner are no better with meats, bread, pasta and rice. The majority of the food you eat is acid forming in the body. You eat without thinking of the dire consequences an acidic diet has on your health. The reason for this is that no one has explained what acid-alkaline balance is and how excessive amounts of acid forming foods and beverages can harm you.

Anything you eat or drink, as well as the air you breathe, leaves an ash in your body. Depending upon its mineral composition, this ash can be either acid, neutral or alkaline waste. When you eat too many acidic foods, your body must compensate by using its alkaline mineral reserves. These reserves are there to buffer the excess acid that is building in your system. You also take medications that may create toxicity, are very stressed, don't exercise enough, don't drink an adequate amount of mineralized water and may have bad posture. All these things make you acidic and toxic.

Many of you have been overly acidic since you were children, possibly beginning in your mother's womb. I remember as an eight or nine-year old child having heel spurs, dry cracked bleeding feet and severe hives all over my body. It occurred at the same time I had a very emotional event occur and was very stressed from having to take a series of school tests. Stress is severely acid forming and damaging to your health. At that time no one could connect my being stressed, dehydrated and acidic to my heel spurs and skin problems. As a young boy I remember having severe heartburn, I would cross my arms over my chest with my eyes closed tight, hoping the intense burning in my chest would stop. That same year I gained an enormous amount of weight in one summer, my breasts were very sensitive and I also began to stutter a lot. I was severely overly acidic and toxic.

Mineral Reserves

For most of my life I made choices that instead of giving me health made me acidic, depleting my tissues of alkalizing minerals. The body stores alkaline forming minerals; in your skin, bones, teeth, muscles and organs. These minerals can be used when needed during future bouts of over acidity. Minerals that are alkaline are Calcium, Magnesium, Sodium, Potassium, Iron and Manganese. They bind and buffer acid forming minerals in the body. Acid forming minerals are Phosphorous, Sulphur, Chlorine, Iodine, Bromine, Fluorine, Copper and Silicon.

For vibrant cellular health we need to have large reserves of alkaline forming minerals. They need the ability to circulate through the tissues to buffer acid that is building in and around the cells. By not having enough alkaline forming minerals from fruits and vegetables, and consuming too many acid forming minerals from highly acidic diets, you become severely acidic, toxic and congested which can lead to most of your health problems.

To regain your health you need to bring your body fluids and especially tissues back into balance. It is extremely important to replenish your body's mineral reserves every day. When you eat a greener diet, including more vegetables and fruits, you begin to replenish important mineral reserves. When we eat, minerals left after digestion are stored for later use in the body. Building up an alkaline mineral reserve through diet changes alone, may take some time.

In addition to a greener diet, adding nutritional products that alkalize and re-mineralize your body will help bring you back to balance faster. When you are more alkaline you feel more energetic with a renewed zeal for life. This can happen in as little as a few days or a few weeks depending on your health. Your body functions better with alkaline minerals, fruits and vegetables are rich in alkalizing minerals. You will find some nutritional help in Chapter Fourteen. The key is using lymphatic activation to get these minerals to circulate around and into your cells.

Looking in the Wrong Place

For the most part medical tests use your blood to monitor pH levels, yet this test is rarely performed. This method is useful to see if the blood is becoming more acidic, but does not tell us if the tissues are overly acidic. Unfortunately, by the time your blood becomes severely acidic you have already been toxic and sick for a long time. Your heart depends on your arterial blood pH to be at a near constant 7.37 - 7.43. Small variations of the blood pH will affect your heart with palpitations or arrhythmias. Large fluctuations could possibly kill you with a heart attack.

The blood will leach minerals from your skin, muscles, bones, teeth or organs to buffer excess acid in the blood in order to keep the heart working optimally. This leaching of minerals is the real cause of osteoporosis. The blood is stealing minerals from your bones to buffer excess acid in your body, which weakens the bone. Most of my patients with osteoporosis, some as young as 30 years old, had no idea how osteoporosis develops and that being overly acidic was a major contributing factor. Occasionally urine is used to test for acidosis but the results are not considered reliable. In Chapter Thirteen we will discuss the relationship between urine and saliva pH testing. Over the past few years I have collected hundreds of pH tests and have realized why urine pH tests are unreliable. It has to do with acid storing in your tissues and not making it into the urine.

You Have Nothing to Lose But Your Health Problems

In September of 2003 my muscles were tight and at times I would have trouble holding onto a glass or signing my name to a check. I was severely lactose intolerant, had life long bowel problems, had been nauseous for six years, and was beginning to suffer with painful hemorrhoids. Brown growths popped out on my left temple and dime sized bald spots kept appearing in the left side of my beard. I would bloat for days from the excess gas in my system. My relatives would tease me by saying I looked pregnant. I remember telling my wife I felt so sick that I felt like I was getting cancer.

Once I learned about acid-alkaline balance and addressed my severe tissue acidosis, all of my problems left. In less than 30 days of eating fruits and vegetables, exercising, taking a few alkalizing products and systemic enzymes I was no longer nauseous, bloated or lactose intolerant and my stomach problems ceased to exist. I lost over 30 pounds and had energy again. Now I did go extreme which is hard for most people. My diet was fruits and vegetables for thirty days, no meat, chicken, fish or grains. My symptoms begin to return when I become more acidic.

Balancing your pH is not something you do once and you're healed. It is something you learn to do everyday at almost every meal. You have nothing to lose by trying a healthier lifestyle for two weeks to 30 days. Armed with the right information you will be able to make the right choices for improved health and a better life.

Being Overly Acidic Slows Your Lymph Flow

Most people are unaware of the importance of the lymphatic system. It is a network of very fine vessels, that can be as thin as a strand of hair to barely visible to the naked eye. This tiny plumbing system must be able to move the excess fluid, acidic waste, large proteins and toxins out of your tissues through lymph vessels and lymph nodes back to your heart to re-enter the blood supply to be cleaned by your organs.

To be very clear, when you are overly acidic your lymphatic system and surrounding tissues constrict from the harsh environment. This limits your circulation creating congestion of acidic waste, proteins, hormones, cholesterol and toxins around and in your cells. In doing research for this book I realized that many of our health problems have to do with excess fluid. This buildup of waste can lead to excess fluid in your tissues affecting all systems of the body.

Here's proof that we are missing the lymphatic systems role in disease. Many of our diseases have symptoms that include excess fluid, i.e. swelling, tumors or fluid filled cysts. Some of these ailments are edema of the limbs, infant and adult hydrocephalus (excess fluid in the cranium), fluid in the ears, swollen prostate, breast cysts, ovarian cysts, swollen lymph nodes, heart failure (excess fluid on the heart), enlarged heart, enlarged spleen, cirrhosis of the liver (fluid filled cysts in liver), polycystic kidney disease, polycystic lung disease, thyroid goiter (enlarged thyroid), water on the knee, ganglion cyst, bursitis and boils. The lymphatic system is responsible for a portion of the blood and waste that does not make it into the veins. When you are overly acidic your lymphatic system constricts and you fill with proteins, fluid and waste. It's a major problem that tissue acidosis, as well as the lymphatic system are not accurately understood in our understanding of disease.

Acid Is Damaging Your Cells

Acid will burn your skin. Think of what would happen if you spilled vinegar, an acid with a pH of 3, on an open cut. It would burn and hurt. The vinegar would be burning and damaging the live cells in the open cut. This is similar to what is happening inside your body. In an acidic environment the cells that make up your lymph and blood vessels, nerves, bones, muscles, organs and tissues are being damaged and destroyed. Heart disease or vascular disease could actually be the result of acidic wastes building in and damaging the tissue of the heart or blood vessels causing inflammation and fibrosis (scarring from protein buildup). Whether your body has low acid for many years or high acid over a shorter period of time, they both negatively impact your health. Even being too alkaline is dangerous, though this is rarely seen. Achieving the right balance is the key.

In the past few decades many books have been written by brilliant men and women who have M.D.'s, N.D.'s and Ph.D.'s addressing the acid-alkaline balance theory. All agree that disease begins when your pH becomes out of balance or overly acidic. I believe we have to look one step further, that acid's affect on our lymphatic system is the "Missed Root Cause of Disease." Once we acknowledge that toxicity in our tissues is the beginning of disease, we will finally be able to address the real cause of most of our current diseases, stagnant fluids that cause protein buildup.

CHAPTER TWO

Acid-Alkaline Balance Theory: A Better Name - Balanced Life Theory

The acid-alkaline balance theory is simple, your body functions best when in balance which is 7 or neutral on the pH scale. When you exhaust your alkaline mineral reserves from your tissues you become overly acidic which is below 7 on the pH scale. This creates an imbalanced acidic internal environment that limits your cellular and overall health. This concept simplifies our medical paradigm of treating 100's of diseases differently. The basis of most disease starts with over acidity or more technically, "tissue acidosis." Instead of treating symptoms of acidosis, such as cancer, heart disease, diabetes, depression and obesity, we would treat or address the underlying cause, an acid or alkaline imbalance that has slowed the lymphatic system creating excess protein in the body. I believe a better name for this acid-alkaline balance theory is a Balanced Life Theory. It's more about balancing your whole life rather than just your diet. This balancing act results in a balanced inner environment and a healthier, happier you.

Balance In and Around Your Cells

Most of you have learned about homeostasis, or being in balance, during high school. It's a very simple principle. Your body is always teetering, moving between an acidic or alkaline pH, trying to be in balance or neutral. Now that I understand acidosis I realize that I was severely out of balance, which was making me sick and overweight. Because of our excessive acidic diets, shallow breathing, daily stress, lack of exercise, constant dehydration and bad posture our cellular environment has become out of balance and toxic. This toxic acidosis makes your internal environment hostile to your cells. The cells will either become damaged, die or mutate to live in the toxic anaerobic (lacking oxygen) environment. This is how diseases like candida and cancer manifest. Every part of your body is made up of cells, including your blood, skin, bones, muscles, and organs. Most of these cells are alive and dependent on blood to receive nutrition and oxygen. Equally important, since they are alive, these cells need to get rid of their own metabolic waste. When you are acidic, your body's ability to nourish as well as clean up waste from around your trillions of cells is compromised. This leads to increased levels of acidic waste, toxins and protein rich fluid in your tissues that limits the flow of interstitial fluid (fluid around your cells), lymph and blood. This congestion in any part of the body is how the disease process begins.

Genetics or Lifestyle Choices

Many experts agree that one third of your health is dependent on genetics. The other two thirds are related to your lifestyle choices. Consequently, it all comes down to the fact that a large number of your own lifestyle choices have made you acidic, tight, overweight or sick. Our wellness center specializes in pain and stress relief. Some of the patients I see have a hard time believing that the majority of their pain and stress is from their diet and lifestyle choices. Outside influences such as environmental toxins, trauma and surgery can cause pain. This undetected tissue acidosis is causing more pain and discomfort by tightening the body, limiting circulation and keeping the initial injury from healing. By making better choices to balance the body, pain is lessened and healing can begin to take place. Healing is all about good, complete circulation.

Balance Your Vices

When you take dangerous drugs like crystal meth, cocaine and heroine your body quickly becomes acidic and toxic. Meth addicts loose their teeth due to extreme acidity and lack of circulation to the gums and nerves of the teeth. Recreational drugs such as alcohol, beer, wine, marijuana and cigarettes are harmful for your tissues, organs and brain. Part of the high you feel is the body reacting to the new toxic environment damaging the cells, constricting your tissues and limiting circulation. Your body is very adaptive and can function for a while with the added poisons you choose. As toxicity builds in the tissues and organs, your circulation and health begin to decline.

We all need ways to unwind and relax. People will continue to use alcohol, tobacco or marijuana. It's very important to realize that even with a small amount of these items you are negatively affecting your body by slowing your circulation. We all need ways to unwind and relax. People will continue to use alcohol, tobacco or marijuana. It's very important to realize that even with a small amount of these items you are negatively affecting your body by slowing your circulation. When you use these recreational drugs to relax you are setting yourself to be more stressed the next day because you are making yourself more acidic. If you are going to use these recreational drugs (alcohol included) you need to understand balance. When using these drugs more than socially, it is very hard to balance their negative side affects. I believe that as a society these vices will always be around. The difficult part is balancing the poisonous affects they have on your body. Too often I hear of someone who stopped drinking or smoking for a decade but still died of cancer. Drinking and smoking create acidity and fibrosis (a buildup of protein, dead cells and fibrin) in the body, when they stop their vice most people don't do anything to remove the acid or fibrosis that is limiting circulation.

Following some of the steps in this book can be a good beginning. Massage, lymphatic activation, manual detoxification, nutritional supplements, extra mineralized water and exercise is all very important to try and balance your vices and to eliminate fibrosis. If you don't exercise to increase circulation, the alcohol, marijuana or cigarettes can make your tissues and organs acidic and constricted. This makes you more toxic and will limit your health. If you are going to drink and smoke; try and Balance it!

Circulation Not Magic

Most of my patients feel results within a few sessions. Many have seen their problems go away after activating their lymphatic system in their first session. Often during an initial session I hear patients say they feel parts of their body tingling or coming alive. Many have had years of pain and are on major doses of pain medications, but after a few sessions of increasing their circulation they are much better. This isn't magic; it's science! By enhancing lymph and blood flow, we increase circulation and detoxification which brings nutrients and oxygen to your cells creating a better internal environment. These patients, because of their pain, are often disabled and very sedentary. After a few sessions of activating lymph flow and increasing circulation, these patients are feeling much better as a result of removing excess toxic fluid, acidic waste and proteins from their tissues.

As they begin to feel better, they become more active. Many patients have said, "I feel alive again." Increased circulation changes the cellular environment to a more alkaline and nourishing environment, helping the cells to begin working optimally. Severe problems such as pain and depression can have vicious cycles that are affected by your lifestyle choices and acidity. These cycles can be broken if you learn what is necessary to alkalize your internal body and increase your circulation to rid your body of excess acid, toxins and proteins. Very often the patient feels so good that they neglect to come in for maintenance. Since many of them remain on their acidic diets, maintain an inactive lifestyle and don't keep up with some type of monthly maintenance for their body, acidic waste and proteins begin to build in the tissues again. This slows the lymph flow and blood circulation. The body becomes more acidic, tight and soon their symptoms begin to return. I joke with some patients that they take better care of their car or home than they do of their own body. They all laugh but it's true. You think you don't have the time to take care of yourself. The sad part is that if you don't maintain your body it will break down.

Patient Profile: Bridget B.

When I first saw Bridget she stood bent over due to the pain in her lower back and left hip. She had battled pain in the area for many years and was barely able to keep it under control. Occasional flare-ups had her bedridden for days. The last few months prior to our meeting had been the worst for her. She could not move without severe pain and she cried often from the pain and desperation she felt. She was on pain medications and she had moved a lounge chair into the kitchen so that she could work for a few minutes at the sink or stove and then lay in her lounge chair to take the pressure off her back.

When I met Bridget I could see the pain in her face and I could see how the pain had gripped her body and was pulling her over. After the first combined session of CranioSacral Therapy and Lymph Drainage Therapy to open her body and enhance her circulation, Bridget wasn't sure she felt any better. I told her to look for small, subtle changes. The next day she came in and said she may be feeling a little less pain. Immediately following her second session, Bridget was sore and barely able to make it to a waiting room chair before she broke down in tears and sobbed from her pain. As she composed herself she explained how she has been crying a lot over the past few months. Before our sessions began Bridget was scheduled to see her doctor within four days for a cortisone injection to try and relieve the pain. She asked me if she should cancel the injection. Without hesitation I said that I couldn't tell her what to do. The decision would be between her and her doctor. I did tell her that she still had three days to find out if we could alleviate some of her pain, then she would be able to make a more informed decision.

After a few sessions Bridget eventually cancelled the appointment for her injection. In one of our earlier sessions I asked Bridget how she was doing and she said that she was seeing a little more improvement. I then asked her if she was still crying a lot. With a smile, she answered no not at all. She was slowly regaining her strength, her pain was decreasing and she was feeling much better mentally. Her face had a smile and she was excited to be getting her life back. She had hope again. After four sessions to ease her pain we did a series of Lymphatic Cellular Detox Massage to increase whole body circulation. In a matter of three days Bridget became severely acidic due to the toxins being released. As a result, she felt tight, weak and sick. By the end of the three days she had dark circles under her eyes and dry skin, but her pain was almost gone. Bridget's back and hip felt their best after the three sessions to drain her body of acidic waste and proteins.

After a few weeks of therapy, when I saw Bridget again she had a bounce in her step. She was standing straighter and she was excited about getting better. Her lounge chair was no longer in the kitchen, she was able to do grocery shopping without an electric cart and she was doing yard work again. She does have her ups and downs but overall she was better. For over a month I saw Bridget get her life back. Then I saw her pain return as our sessions became less frequent, but not to the extreme level as when I first met her. She was filling with waste again. As the pain increased Bridget received three cortisone injections but still had her pain. She was hoping the injections would be a magic bullet to stop her pain. She only saw a minor improvement in her pain level for a short period of time after the injection; overall she was disappointed with the results. When pain or symptoms return, I tell patients to examine their choices over the past few days or weeks. Did they experience increased stress, eat more acidic foods, become dehydrated or refrain from exercising. After speaking with Bridget I learned she had made no real changes in her diet, which is high in acid foods and she was not exercising.

After a few months of just controlling Bridget's pain I suggested she try another series of the Cellular Detoxification Massage to increase detoxification in order to alleviate more of her pain. She was reluctant. After three consecutive sessions (one hour three days in a row) of increasing her circulation she was remarkably better again. After seeing her pains disappear after the first detoxification, and then once again this time, she became a believer. Bridget now understood that acid and excess proteins are something she has to learn to manage if she wants to keep her pain from getting out of control. To help control acid, Bridget started taking an alkalizing product and began exercising. She has learned to stretch and do specific exercises daily to keep her problem area open and circulating. Every four to six weeks Bridget comes in for a detox session to help keep her circulation open. Every few months she does a few sessions consecutively to deeply clean her body. Bridget now realizes she has to control her pH and circulation in order to control her pain. She has told me that her daily walking is what is making the difference especially adding two-forty second sprints of walking faster every other day.

Signs of Being Overly Acidic

You have always been aware of the signs of over acidity; you just didn't realize that being too acidic was the cause. For example, we have all had an acquaintance that could only wear certain jewelry because inexpensive jewelry would turn their skin green. The jewelry is not to blame; their skin is so acidic it is reacting with the metal creating a chemical reaction that turns their skin green. If your skin turns green from jewelry, check your saliva and urine pH. You may be overly acidic and toxic. Some signs of over acidity are: acne, aggression, stuttering, tight or sore muscles, fatigue, dizziness, allergies, multiple chemical sensitivities, eczema, hair loss, panic attacks, anxiety, depression, menstrual cramps, infertility, sore breasts, low sex drive, esophageal gastric reflux disease, bloating, heartburn, diarrhea, constipation, TMJ dysfunction, headaches, migraines, inability to think clearly, sinus problems, dark rings under the eyes, pale complexion and an irregular heartbeat, to name only a few.

Lung and Kidney Function Help Maintain Blood pH

According to the Merck Manual your lungs and kidneys help balance blood pH by removing acid waste from the body. I believe this is important to note given that many of your diseases occur in the lungs and kidneys. Can being overly acidic overwhelm your lungs and kidneys and cause diseases like asthma, emphysema, lung or kidney cancer or polycystic kidney disease?

I have seen many patients who have asthma or emphysema who have never smoked. Today more people who have never smoked are being diagnosed with lung cancer. Your lungs convert carbonic acid to CO2 (carbon dioxide) and water. The simple act of breathing can help alter your blood pH, so deep breathing throughout the day is extremely important. If you look around many people rarely deep breath, this is especially true if you are concentrating on something like the computer or paying bills. Your kidneys excrete either acid or base (alkaline) to alter your blood pH. At our wellness center most patients have low back pain in addition to tightness in other areas. Your kidneys are in the low back. As they become congested with excess acid and proteins, they become more toxic and begin to tighten, affecting the surrounding tissues in the low back.

One important point to make is that the lymphatic system is responsible for collecting and moving acidic waste out of the tissues, back to the heart and blood supply and then to the kidneys, lungs and other organs. When your lymphatic system slows because you are acidic, the entire process of removing acidic wastes and proteins from around your cells and out of your organs is compromised. I believe this leads to toxicity and congestion in the tissues and organs which can reduce organ function and lead to inflammation and diseases such as pancreatitis, meningitis, cirrhosis of the liver, kidney stones, gall stones, enlarged prostate or spleen.

It's Not Old Age

Acid is stealing your lives. Recently while at a health fair for seniors I was amazed at how many of the seniors are shaking, bent over or twisted from their tight muscles. Some individuals look as if they are actually turning to stone as their membranes around their organs and brain becomes tighter and tighter due to acidity and proteins building in their tissues. When you are overly acidic your body is tight and we feel less mobile. This generation consumes a large amount of acid in the form of meats, eggs, bread, and coffee. We all have relatives who as they age start having more aches and pains, muscle tightness, high blood pressure, shakiness or lack of energy. Don't blame it on old age, they are becoming more acidic and toxic.

I have many acquaintances that are between 70 and 90 who have pain from tight muscles, sciatica, shingles or arthritis. These problems are all caused by over acidity and a lack of circulation. Their pain has stopped them from doing things they loved to do. They may have been simple things that they enjoyed, like gardening, shopping, crocheting or playing cards, but now the pain makes them less mobile. You must be open-minded and at least consider whether your medications, acidic diets, inactivity and dehydration and posture might be making you have more pain or a lack of energy. It would only take a few weeks of applying the information within this book to change your life dramatically. I am amazed at how often I hear people in their 40's and 50's complain about their aches and pains and then laugh, saying it must be old age. It's not old age, it's acidosis that is tightening their body. Old age shouldn't hurt. It should be a special time when you get to enjoy your life and not worry about losing your mind or health. Many seniors are having health concerns due to over acidity that is limiting their life.

Acid-Alkaline Food Chart - A Partial Hope

The reason we don't have better health is because we don't have the right information. There are many acid-alkaline food charts in books and on the Internet, some may conflict slightly. Why are we unaware of what foods make us healthy and which foods, when eaten in abundance, can limit our circulation and make us sick? For example, even though milk is neutral on the pH scale, the large amount of protein in cow's milk meant to fatten a calf, may add to your existing protein and congestion problems.

When you sprout seeds and grains they become more alkaline. Most fresh vegetable and fruit juices are highly alkaline. Homemade vegetable broth is an extremely alkalizing beverage. Essentially fruits, vegetables and some grains are alkaline and everything else is acid. I believe there will be confusion regarding which foods and products are acid and which are alkaline forming in our body. The only way to make it less confusing is for every farmer, rancher or producer of anything we eat, drink, smoke, put on our skin or hair, be required to test and assign a pH value to their product. This one step of showing pH values on packages will simplify our ability to balance the acid and alkaline in our lives.

ALKALIZING FOODS

VEGETABLES:

Alfalfa
Asparagus
Barley Grass
Beets
Broccoli
Brussel Sprouts
Cabbage
Carrot
Cauliflower
Celery
Chard
Chlorella
Collard Greens
Cucumber
Dulce
Dandelions
Edible Flowers
Eggplant
Fermented Veggies
Garlic
Kale
Fermented Veggies
Lettuce
Mushrooms
Mustard Greens
Onions
Parsnips
Peas
Peppers
Pumpkin
Rutabaga
Sea Vegetables
Spirulina
Sprouts
Squashes
Watercress
Wheat Grass

ORIENTAL VEGETABLES:

Maitake	Shitake	Nori
Daikon	Kombu	Umeboshi
Dandelion Root	Reishi	Wakame

FRUITS:

Apple	Grapes	Peach
Apricot	Grapefruit	Pear
Avocado	Lime	Fresh Pineapple
Banana	Honeydew	All Berries
Cantaloupe	Melons	Tangerine
Cherries	Nectarine	Tomato
Currants	Lemon	Tropical Fruits
Dates/Figs	Orange	Watermelon

SEEDS & NUTS:

Almonds	Millet	Sunflower Seeds
Chestnuts	Pumpkin Seeds	Sprouted Seeds
Flax Seeds		

SPICES & SEASONINGS:

Chili Pepper	Ginger	Sea Salt
Cinnamon	Miso	Tamari
Curry	Mustard	Most Herbs

NEUTRAL or NEAR NEUTRAL FOODS

Organic Milk	Soft Cheeses	Butter

Even though milk and dairy products may be close to neutral they are full of proteins that are meant to make a calf 500 pounds within one year. These large proteins can add to congestion and mucus formation in your body.

ACIDIFYING FOODS

ANIMAL PROTEIN:

Beef	Mussels	Shrimp
Clams	Oysters	Scallops
Fish	Pork	Tuna
Lamb	Rabbit	Turkey
Lobster	Salmon	Venison

FRUITS:

Cranberries

GRAINS:

Amaranth	Oats (rolled)	Spelt
Barley	Quinoa	Wheat
Buckwheat	Rice Cakes	Wheat Cakes
Corn	Rice (all)	White Flour
Kamut	Rye	

Most grains are acid forming. Whole grains and grains such as Buckwheat, Kamut, Millet and Brown Rice may not be alkaline, but they have more nutritional value than processed white grains. Quinoa (pronounced keenwa) is not really a grain, but a seed from a plant similar to spinach. It can be used as a grain, contains high levels of easily digestible protein and is very nutritious.

NUTS & BUTTERS:

Cashews	Peanuts	Peanut Butter
Pecans	Walnuts	

DRUGS & CHEMICALS:

Chemical	Herbicides	Pesticides
Recreational Drugs	Medicinal & Psychedelic	

ALCOHOL:

Beer	Wine	Hard Liquor

CHAPTER THREE

Saliva and Urine pH Study Results – There is a Major Problem!

When I first learned about acidosis from Dr. Desgrey, he told me he had been testing the saliva pH of people he met for a long time and that most people he tested were overly acidic. I knew my family and I were severely acidic but I was curious to see for myself how many people were toxic from an acidic pH. I started an informal study, asking patients if they would self-test their saliva pH and give me their pH results. Over 100 people shared their saliva pH test results with me, at that time only a few individuals tested in a healthy range of 6.5 to 7.5 on the pH scale. I remember being amazed that the majority of people were just about 5.5 on the pH scale. This is a very acidic and toxic environment for your cells.

It's important to note that the pH strips I was using at the time only went as low as 5.5. When I started using a pH test strip that went as low as 5.0, many people started testing at 5.0 or 5.1. I realized then that there was a major problem. Your saliva and urine pH should test between 6.5 and 7.5. Many people are testing at 5.0, which is 100 times more acidic than 7.0 or neutral. This undetected acidosis is hurting you by constricting and corroding your inner body. When I was a teenager I worked in a gas station, when battery acid got on my clothes those areas touched by acid would corrode and fall apart in a short matter of time. Acidic urine at 5.0 is not as dangerous as battery acid with a pH of 0.5, but over years or decades a pH of 5.0 in any part if the body could slowly corrode, constrict and damage your skin, muscles, bones, organs or central nervous system.

I spent months calling doctors at the National Institutes of Health to see who I could tell about this undetected toxic tissue acidosis. The National

Institutes of Health is not one organization. It is made up of many doctors and researchers spread across our nation in different universities or hospitals. It is a fractured organization. Often one department does not know what the other is doing. Many doctors I spoke with didn't know who to refer me to, or would say they aren't studying acidosis or the lymphatic system. One NIH researcher actually said to me, "How could a large part of our population be severely acidic and we (the medical community) don't know about it?"

I never anticipated being an acid-alkaline researcher. On the advice of two doctors at the NIH, I began to collect data to prove there is a problem. I first started a formal study of saliva pH. I began collecting and documenting the data from over 100 individuals, mostly patients, who self-tested their saliva pH and gave me their data. If this study is any indication of the health of our nation, then as much as 90% of our nation may be acidic, and more than 43% may be severely acidic and sick! There is a devastating national problem that is making us ill and few are aware of it. It is also a global problem! Most countries consume white rice, white flour products, meats, chicken, fish, coffee, tea, alcohol and smoke. All of these are very acid forming in the body.

Documented Saliva pH Study

The objective of the study was simple: to collect data on the saliva pH of a portion of our population. The participants were mostly patients who already had health problems. They fasted for two hours and were shown how to use and read a simple pH test strip accurately. After they self-tested their saliva pH, someone familiar with reading pH test strips verified their results for accuracy. The following are results from 103 Participants:

Saliva pH Test Results 103 Participants

Severe Acidosis (5.0 - 5.4)	45	43.6%
Unhealthy (5.5 - 5.9)	27	26.2%
Slightly Acidic (6.0 - 6.4)	24	23.3%
Healthy Saliva pH Range (6.5 - 7.5)	7	6.8%

When I saw that over 90% of those tested were outside of a healthy pH range and as many as 43% in our study were severely acidic, I knew there was a problem. You don't have to be a medical researcher to see there may be a major undetected acidosis negatively affecting our nation.

A Significant Study

To show you the significance of this study, let me tell you about a meeting I had with David Whelan the President of Phion Inc., a pH test strip and supplement company that is based on the Internet. I had the results from my study and I wanted to discuss them with someone familiar with pH. A point that needs to be made is that at that time, Phion's pH test strip only went as low as 5.5. When I showed David the study results that over 43% of those tested were below 5.0. he thought for a moment and then said he gets calls from customers across the nation saying the test strip isn't working. You see, in my study 43% of the participants tested below 5.5 and if the person using the test strip is below 5.5 the strip does not change color. This looks as though the pH strip is not working. Actually, they were just too acidic to register a reading.

The fact that this web based company had been receiving calls about the strips not working further validates that there is a major problem of over acidity in our nation, possibly the world. I told David that I believe some people will test below 5.0. He understood the importance of my study and spent a great deal of time and money to lower his pH test strip from 5.5 to 4.5.

Wickenburg pH Health Study

In 2007 I started the Wickenburg, Arizona pH Health Study. Wickenburg is a beautiful, old west town around 45 minutes outside of Phoenix. I wanted to have data from urine and saliva pH tests from a more general segment of the population rather than my patients who tended to already have headaches, migraines, chronic fatigue, fibromyalgia, MS, cancer or have pain. We had 150 participants, who read about the study in the local paper and volunteered to participate. They fasted for two hours, self-tested their saliva and urine pH and had the results verified by someone familiar with reading pH tests. We collected the pH data and what we found was very different from our first study using only data from saliva pH tests of patients. The following are the results:

Wickenburg pH Health Study		Saliva	Urine
Severe Acidosis	(5.0 - 5.4)	3%	51%
Unhealthy	(5.5 - 5.9)	12%	22%
Slightly Acidic	(6.0 - 6.4)	37%	10%
Healthy Saliva pH Range	(6.5 - 7.5)	46%	11%
Too Alkaline	(8.0 - above)	2%	6%

General Population pH Results

In the Wickenburg pH health study the individuals we collected data from were a good representation of what you would find in a more senior community in any small town in America. Their ages ranged from the 20's to 90's, some were healthy some were not. In the urine pH results over 80% were outside of a healthy pH, while over 50% were severely acidic, probably 100 times more acidic than they should be testing. Many of these individuals had no idea that they should be balancing their internal body to reach 7, or neutral on the pH scale.

In the Wickenburg saliva testing we saw fewer individuals (3%) with severe pH than the first saliva pH study (43%). I believe the reason for the difference was that the first saliva pH study used data from patients who were already very sick and toxic, that's why their saliva tested severely acidic. In the Wickenburg pH Study data was taken from a part of the general population where the acidity had not reached such severe levels in the saliva.

Detoxification

According to the Merriam-Webster Dictionary, detoxify means to remove a poison or toxin. The poison in this case is the toxic, acidic cellular waste in your tissues. Herbs, diet and bodywork such as massage, have been used to detoxify the body and organs for thousands of years. However, if areas in the body are already overly acidic, tight and congested, as in cancer or fibromyalgia, then circulation through the tissues is slowed or impeded. Subsequently, supplements, herbs, massage, even medications, such as chemotherapy drugs or arthritis drugs may not get deeply into these walled off areas of congested, toxic, tissue efficiently.

At the Lymphatic Wellness Center we use a series of sessions to gently activate the lymphatics to improve circulation and detoxification in the tissues and organs. Whole body lymphatic activation helps to rid the body of acidic waste and toxins by gently by increasing circulation to help remove fibrosis and sclerosis (a buildup of proteins like fibrin and cellular waste). Lymphatic Cellular Detox Massage is designed to gently, manually activate the lymphatics very efficiently and deeply, including in the tissues, muscles, bones, organs and membranes that surround the brain and spinal cord. Over time improved circulation makes your entire body less toxic, more alkaline and promotes a much healthier environment for your cells to live and thrive in. Most patients see and feel a difference in the first week or two after lymphatic activation.

Same Reactions Over And Over

During a series of Lymphatic Cellular Detox Massages patients schedule five to six sessions over a three to four week period. The first two sessions are a week apart to slowly begin the process of activating the lymph. In the second or third week the patient comes in for a one hour session to activate the lymphatics on three consecutive days. The three days in a row allows for a much deeper detox than if the patient were to come in for weekly sessions. Patients have felt many of the same detox reactions over the course of their sessions.

After years of storing acidic waste and proteins your first lymphatic activation session may make you feel sick, tired, have problems sleeping, digestion problems, more pain and discomfort for a day. This is when some individuals will have some reaction to the detoxification. Some individuals may only feel some fatigue for a day while others will feel their worst fatigue, pain, anxiety or depression. In subsequent sessions most patients only feel a little fatigue, while others have new found energy and clarity from the start. Below I detail what patients have felt during their three consecutive sessions.

Day One: Immediately following their first session of the three on consecutive days, patients will initially feel more relaxed. Later in the day some will feel more tired, achy and will have a restless night sleep. During the session we are manually releasing large amounts of toxic waste and proteins from the tissues and organs that will further congest an already congested body. You see as the lymphatics are activated waste is collected and must return to the heart and through all the organs to be eliminated from the kidneys, lungs and skin. The tissues and organs will congest because of the excess waste, proteins and toxins released into the system. I tell patients that if they are tired and feel the need to lie down for a nap, first do something to move their circulation in order to help move the toxins out of their system. That can start with drinking water, then some deep breathing exercises, light exercise, walking or a hot bath with Epsom salts. Your urine will become more cloudy or dark as wastes are leaving your body. Eating lightly and drinking extra water throughout the day is very important. Eating too heavy or being dehydrated can further clog your system and intensify your detox reaction.

Day Two: Remember this work is very light. Many patients have come into the second session saying they felt like a train hit them. They have a headache, no energy, stomach problems and they just feel lousy. Excess acid waste in your body is not good for you. After activating their lymph flow, some patients will feel better for a while after the session. As more acid waste and proteins enter and congests their system, they will begin to feel more tired, emotional, cranky, angry, aggressive, sore, anxious or depressed. I now know that during a lymphatic activation session whatever your usual problems are, they will be intensified for a day or two as congestion and toxicity increases in the body. Most had a horrible night's sleep the second night. For years I had wondered why so many of my patients had problems with insomnia. Now I know that people who don't sleep well are overly acidic, protein filled and toxic.

Day Three: Most patients will wake up on day three feeling drained but better. The circulation in their body is less overwhelmed with acidic waste. They come to their third session weak but smiling, able to joke at how sick they felt the day before. It is no joke. Excess acid and proteins are slowly damaging your cells and negatively affecting your physical and mental health. Most patients will begin to have much more energy, less pain and sleep better than they did prior to the sessions. Over the past few years, almost on a daily basis, I have seen the positive effects people feel after lymphatic activation. I am a true believer in the fact that over acidity and its negative affect on the lymphatic system is slowly killing you and severely hurting children!

Human Guinea Pig

In writing this book I wanted to experiment with detoxification on myself, so I could experience its effects. I stopped taking my alkalizing products and ate more acid forming foods as I did in the past. Within a few days I started feeling bloated in my abdomen and experienced minor muscle tightness in my body. After approximately one week I started noticing some increasing muscle tightness in my low back, upper shoulders and neck, a slight headache, gas, and I was itchier. By the second week I started having a stabbing pain in my right shoulder as I raised my arm. By the next day I could barely move my arm. By the end of the day every time I tried to use my arm I was getting sharp pains in my shoulder and chest, behind my heart. This actually frightened my wife and I.

I decided to stop my experiment; I wasn't willing to risk my health any further. I did learn that when you detox your body and are eating more alkaline foods, when you re-introduce large amounts of acid into the body you feel it very quickly. This happens because you removed acid waste and proteins, making your body less congested, toxic and healthier. When you are in balance and less congested and introduce more acid back to your body, you will actually feel the tissues tighten due to the toxicity of the cellular environment.

The stabbing pain in my chest and sore arm concerned me enough to go to the doctor the next day in order to rule out any heart problems. By this time my arm was useless to me. Anytime I tried to move it, even a little, the pain would be excruciating. After my doctor looked at my x-rays' she said I was fine. I had some inflammation from calcium deposits in the shoulder and an irritation in the muscles behind my heart. She prescribed a sling for my arm and if the pain increased she recommended I take an anti-inflammatory. She said I might not be able to return to work for a few weeks.

Calcium deposits are very common in our population. We get them on our spine, teeth, shoulders, heels, fingers and on our head. I have always thought calcium deposits were the body's mechanism to protect an area by strengthening it with calcium. Now that I understand acidosis, the calcium deposit in my shoulder was calcium being leached out of the tissue or bone to buffer excess acid in the area.

When I went home I started taking alkalizing products throughout the day and decided to eat mostly green for the next few days. When I say green I mean more fruits and vegetables. That night I had to take an anti-inflammatory to relieve some of the increasing pain. Later as the alkalizing products released more acidic waste it began to congest my body. I started becoming very achy, sore, cranky, short-tempered and was starting to feel like I was getting a cold or flu. My wife heated a cup of vegetable broth for me before I went to bed. During the night I had such intense sweats from the detoxification from the supplements we had to change the sheets on the bed twice.

Felt Like the Flu

The next morning I felt horrible, like I had the flu. Some of you may be saying that maybe I did have the flu. No, this is how excess acid and proteins in your system affects your body. Luckily I only had three appointments in the afternoon because I didn't have the energy to get out of bed. After taking alkalizing products and more vegetable broth, I slept all morning. When I woke, I felt drained but better and went to my office early for my appointments. While waiting for my first patient I was pacing between my office and the reception area, I couldn't stop, it was uncontrollable. My mind kept racing from one thought to another. Finally my patient arrived and as we started our session I began to shiver so I put a towel over my shoulders. I tried to concentrate on my patient but my mind was racing and I felt an uncontrollable urge to bolt for the door. It took a lot of focus for me to work with the patient. Finally after twenty minutes I couldn't sit there anymore. I explained how I was feeling and that I had to leave. The patient was a regular patient and was very understanding. When I went out to the reception area I asked my office manager to call and cancel my other appointments. I went home, had more vegetable broth and alkalizing products and then went to bed. The next morning I woke up feeling much better. My healing crisis was over. With continued alkalizing supplements and lymphatic activation, within four days my arm felt good enough that I could go back to work and my chest pain had disappeared. I realized later that I had taken three times the recommended amount for one alkalizing product. It overloaded my system with too much waste and produced a very severe healing crisis. Too much of even good things can be bad for you.

When I was in the office waiting for my patient I couldn't focus my mind or sit still. Now recalling that incident I think of children with ADHD, Asperger's or autism. Some of the children I have seen are always in motion, very hyperactive and aggressive. I wonder if the excess acid and proteins that made me want to pace and kept me from not thinking clearly could be affecting these children as well?

Healing Crisis

When you start lymphatic activation or a detoxification, whether it's using some herbal supplements, eating more fruits and vegetables, getting a few massages, CranioSacral Therapy, Lymph Drainage Therapy or a series of Lymphatic Cellular Detox Massage, you may feel sick before you feel better. It's called a healing crisis. At first as acid wastes and proteins are released from the tissues and enter into the lymphatic system, your lymph vessels and organs become overwhelmed and more acidic. As the body becomes more toxic from excess acidic waste you begin to feel sick. The healing crisis may only last a few hours to a few days. You can alleviate some of the symptoms of a healing crisis by eating a lighter, greener diet, drinking extra mineralized water throughout the day, deep breathing, doing some mild exercise and taking an Epsom salt bath. Epsom salt is magnesium sulfate, combined with the warmth of the bath, it helps to relax your body and increase circulation. For myself and my children I place 2 cups in a large warm bath. For a smaller infant bath I suggest 1/4-1/2 cup. Too much Epsom salt is irritating to the skin.

Slow As You Go

It is important to go through a detoxification slowly. Even eating too many fruits and vegetables or taking too many alkalizing products can create a severe healing crisis. Be careful not to over alkalize. When I inadvertently took three times the dose of one product, it was overwhelming. This will flood your system with excessive amounts of acidic waste that will overload your organs. This congestion can make you very sick. If you are already sick and frail the excess acid and proteins entering your organs may possibly be too much for your system and weaken you further.

If you are pregnant or have health concerns you should always consult with your doctor before lymphatic activation or a detoxification. If you are pregnant you don't need to go through a detoxification just clean up your life-style choices. Over a few weeks slowly start to increase your water intake, cut out processed foods, green-up your diet with fruits and vegetables (mostly veg-etables at first), practice deep breathing, slowly add some non-jarring aerobic exercise and mild strength training. This will help move your lymph flow and blood circulation and slowly detox your tissues and those of the fetus. If you change too much, too quickly the body can become overwhelmed with acid waste and proteins becoming very toxic. This is not healthy for either mother or fetus.

VERY IMPORTANT - During the first few weeks of pregnancy many of the organs of the fetus are being formed. Be extremely careful during this time so as not to create excess waste and toxins, which could create a bad environment for developing fetal cells. Being well hydrated and eating more alkaline are very important in creating a healthy cellular environment for the fetus.

pH / Detoxification Study Using Manual Therapies

I wanted to find out as much as I could about the effects of acidosis on the body. I started a second study to monitor the saliva pH of participants before and after three 60-minute sessions that enhance lymph flow. Over 65 patients received one combined session of Craniosacral Therapy (CST) and Lymph Drainage Therapy (LDT) per day on three consecutive days. Prior to the start of each session, the participants were asked to indicate their pain level, mental well being, energy level and sleep quality by circling a number from 0 to 5 in each category. On the scale 0 was good while 5 was bad. It was amazing to see that over 70% of the participants felt a worsening of their health problems as toxicity rose in their body due to the lymphatic activation. Many experienced increases in pain, fatigue, insomnia, digestive problems and depression after the first or second sessions. As we released more acid waste from their tissues their system would become more acidic and congested, making them feel like they were getting a cold or flu. During the detoxification, a few participants, over 13%, felt some minor fatigue but overall they had no bad side effects to the lymphatic activation. It made them feel better from the first session without a severe detox reaction. A very small group, less than 6%, felt no difference in their health problems after a series of detoxifications. I believe most of this small group, those who felt no difference, are very congested and their circulation is severely impeded. It may take many weeks of multiple sessions of specific therapies such as CranioSacral Therapy, Lymph Drainage Therapy or Lymphatic Cellular Detox Massage and supplements to help detox the tissues to improve circulation. By the end of the series of detoxifications most participants felt their experience was a positive one and felt their health problems had improved.

Aggression, Anxiety, Depression and Cloudy Thinking - Toxic Brain

In general, patients experienced the same reactions from lymphatic activation we discussed earlier. They first felt tired, became cranky, would have insomnia, and more aches and pain. But one thing I heard more than a few times was that they were feeling very aggressive, agitated, anxious, or depressed. Many also said that they felt as if they weren't able to think clearly. After seeing and hearing this over and over, I now believe that being overly acidic, having a malfunctioning lymphatic system and resulting protein buildup plays a major role in anxiety, depression, aggression, bipolar, dementia, Alzheimer's and most of our mental maladies. Later in Chapter Seven I present research that shows the lymphatics play an important role in cerebrospinal fluid and protein reabsorption.

Cerebrospinal fluid helps to nourish, clean and protect the brain, spinal cord and nerves. If you are acidic, your lymphatic system slows, creating congestion in all systems of the body including the brain. If your cerebrospinal fluid becomes acidic, protein filled and toxic it can have a devastating effect on your ability to think as in depression, autism and Alzheimer's. When you feel tight, achy, are getting a headache or can't think clearly, you are becoming more acidic and toxic. This is a sign for you to activate your lymphatic system and rebalance your internal body to improve mental health.

CHAPTER FOUR

Lymph Flow Completes Circulation

Your health depends on many things, but one of the most important is circulation. Proper circulation is how the cells receive nutrition and oxygen as well as rid themselves of their own toxic wastes. When your blood, interstitial fluid (fluid around the cells) and lymph fluid (all these fluids at one time were blood and will return to the blood stream) are circulating optimally, your cells are constantly bathed in a nourishing environment and you feel healthy and alive. When you become to acidic or to alkaline, your lymph flow becomes impeded, limiting blood flow into the tissues or organs. As waste and toxicity build, you begin to feel tired, tight and achy. When you physically check your circulation, you check for a strong pulse in the large arteries in your neck, wrists, top of the feet or behind your knee. There are possibly millions of miles of additional tiny vessels that can congest and affect the health of a certain part of the body.

Whenever I have read about the circulatory system, or have seen posters about circulation, they include the heart, arteries, capillaries and veins. What they don't mention is the lymphatic system and its important roles in completing circulation and maintaining circulation around the cells that make up your tissues. When the lymphatic system is more alkaline it is more efficient in helping to remove excess fluid, waste and proteins from around your cells. A proper functioning lymphatic system is essential in maintaining balance and health in your tissues, skin, muscles, bones, organs and brain.

Circulation Basics

Let's start with the basics. Your blood circulation is a loop of vessels that starts with your heart pumping oxygenated and mineral rich blood down the arteries into smaller and smaller vessels called arterioles. When the blood reaches the tiny arterial side of the capillaries, it moves out into the capillary bed and into the tissue delivering oxygen, nutrients and hormones to your cells. On the venous side of the capillary bed, the veins collect the deoxygenated interstitial fluid (fluid around the cells) full of carbon dioxide, acid waste, proteins and other cellular debris to return it to the heart. As the veins pick up the fluid, 2% to 10% of this fluid, waste and large proteins, are unable to move into the veins and become trapped in the tissues around the cells.

The lymphatic vessels must remove the 2-10% of fluid and debris that is left in the tissues. If this fluid in the tissues was partially blocked to the lymphatics you would have a buildup of carbon dioxide, protein, acidic waste and toxins around your cells. Over time this buildup of cellular waste could make you very toxic and sick as in Candida or cancer. If this leftover fluid between the cells were not picked up by the lymphatic system you would slowly swell to death.

The Lymphatic Systems Beginnings

Insight into the lymphatic system may have begun as far back as Hippocrates (460-377 B.C.) when he spoke of "white blood", used the expression "chyle" and defined a "lymphatic temperament."

In 1622 Gasparo Asselli, an Italian physician and surgeon, observed the white milky veins of a dog. This was the first documented discovery of the lymphatic vessels. The white, milky veins are lymphatic vessels that are transporting fats absorbed during digestion from the intestinal tract. Many researchers before and after Asselli have studied the anatomy of the lymphatic system. It is only recently that we are beginning to understand the lymphatic system's vital role in maintaining health.

In 1920 American physician Earl C. Miller, D.O. published many articles relating to his "Miller thoracic pump technique", which is still in use today. The technique called for gently pumping the thoracic (chest) area. Dr. Miller wrote that his technique is an effective lymphatic pump, which could greatly increase the lymphatic circulation in the whole body. He has written that his thoracic pump technique would help speed the lymphatic absorption of toxins from the body. He believed that there was enough proof in the theory that all infections can be cured by increased lymphatic absorption.

In 1922 Frederick P. Millard, D.O. of Toronto, Ontario published "Applied Anatomy of the Lymphatics". In his book Dr. Millard, with other experts in anatomy, such as Earl. C. Miller, D.O., bring the lymphatic system alive with detailed descriptions. He used the term "lymphatic drainage" to describe his specific work on the lymphatic vessels and nodes.

In 1936, Danish massage practitioner and Dr. of Philosophy Emil Vodder, introduced his new technique Manual Lymph Drainage (MLD). He developed this technique to drain the neck and face to alleviate his patients' sinus and acne problems. He had difficulty proving its effectiveness at the time.

It was not until 1967 that German Physician Johannes Asdonk scientifically tested MLD on 20,000 patients. Over time he established the effectiveness of working with the lymphatic system.

Currently, Bruno Chikly M.D., D.O. (hon), developer of Lymph Drainage Therapy (LDT) studied and improved upon the existing lymph drainage techniques. Dr. Chikly is one of the first to train lymphatic therapists to manually feel the specific rhythm, pressure, quality and direction of the lymph flow. This ability to monitor the river of lymph in the body is important to your health. Advanced therapists can feel and interact with the lymph flow anywhere in the body to help increase circulation through areas that may be congested and toxic.

Lymphatic System Is Overlooked

The lymphatic system is a critical component to your survival. Yet it is not properly recognized in the idea of disease. When this vast network of tiny vessels and nodes are not able to efficiently handle the removal of metabolic waste and excess fluid from your interstitial spaces, your cells become congested and don't function properly. The lymphatic system has major documented roles in maintaining the health of connective tissue, which makes up the majority of the body.

This next statement is from Silent Waves by Dr. Chikly: "part of the constituents of the blood will filter out of the blood capillaries. This blood capillary filtrate will join the surrounding tissues, passing through the interstitial environment (interstitium) - the interstices between each cell, to be further reabsorbed in the lymphatic capillaries. The lymphatic system fine tunes the drainage of the interstitium (connective tissue) and thus constitutes a sort of "overflow" for the water and excess substances in the interstitial environment. In fact, if the lymphatic system did not recover the protein-rich liquid (a large part of which the venous system cannot recover), the body would probably develop major systemic edemas (protein loss), auto-intoxication and die in 24 to 48 hours .... About 75 to 100g of proteins per day can escape from the blood circulation; this is about 50% of the protein circulating in the blood plasma per day. These proteins are transported in the lymphatic vessels."

Large proteins, which have escaped from the blood system and remain in the tissues, are recovered by the lymphatic system. When your lymphatic system is not functioning optimally due to acidity, excess proteins or trauma, cellular waste, germs, toxins and large proteins that have escaped from the blood vessels build in your tissues, including your organs, decreasing circulation. Over time the buildup of waste limits circulation through the tissues or organ and the disease process begins. There are specific diseases such as fatal familial insomnia, batten disease, autism and Alzheimer's that are associated with a buildup of proteins in the brain. The lymphatic system, if working optimally, captures proteins that have escaped into the tissues, organs and brain.

Disease Starts in Stagnant Fluid Around Your Cells

I believe this missed tissue acidosis, and specifically its negative affect on the lymphatic system, is where disease starts, especially in the interstitial spaces (spaces around your cells). In the book "Sick and Tired" by Robert O. Young Ph.D. and his wife Shelley, they write about a Dr. O.C. Gruner and his view that disease starts when intercellular fluid ceases to flow. After further research I learned Dr. Gruner was a Canadian Physician at McGill University in the 1930's and head of the Archibold Cancer Research Committee of Montreal. I believe Dr. Gruner was totally accurate in his description below as to where disease starts. The "pool" or "lake" he mentions is the interstitial fluid (fluid around your cells), "canaliculi" are small canals or vessels and "patent" means to be open.

Dr. Gruner writes "*Unless the outlet of the pool is patent, and the canaliculi likewise, chemical changes take place in the stagnant fluid. Moreover, the parts beyond cease to receive the materials needed... Should this movement be arrested in any part of the body, however small be the site, and however short be the time - what we call "disease" begins... It may be some time before the signs of obstruction become evident... for the surplus capacity of the "lake" is so great... We have this principle then: there is only one disease. All 414 (or so) diseases described in textbooks of medicine are fundamentally forms of one and the same disorder... The problem to be solved in every case of sickness is "for what reason has the flow of intercellular fluid ceased and in what site has it ceased?"...*

Because of its importance I want to clarify the first three sentences. Unless the outlet of the interstitial fluids (fluid around your cells) is open and the vessels also open, chemical changes take place in the stagnant fluid around your cells. Moreover, the parts beyond, deeper in the tissue or organ, stop receiving the materials such as oxygen, nutrition and hormones. Should this movement of fluid be stopped in any part of the body, however small the site and however short the time; what we call disease begins.

One reason for ceased intercellular flow is tissue acidosis, which constricts your lymphatic system, slowing the lymph flow and hindering interstitial fluid from leaving around your cells. This limits the ability of fresh blood to travel deeply into the cells, tissues and organs limiting their function. Over time acid waste builds in your tissues and organs, the stagnant fluid goes through further chemical changes and becomes toxic to your cells. The cells either die or adapt to their hostile environment. Acid and its negative affect on the lymphatic system is the Missed Root Cause of Disease.

According to Dr. Baroody's Alkalize or Die, "The countless names of illnesses do not really matter. What does matter is that they all come from the same root cause...too much tissue acid waste in the body!"

The Key: Over Acidity Slows Lymph Flow

Books on acid-alkaline balance say that disease comes from one imbalance, over acidity. Some even briefly mention acids negative affect on the lymphatic system. What they don't understand is the lymphatic system's true importance in allowing blood to circulate through your tissues and organs.

This next statement is the key to all your health problems. ***When you are overly acidic your lymph flow slows and your tissues and organs become congested with excess proteins.*** The lymphatic system can no longer properly drain the fluid and waste left around your cells and fresh blood cannot pass deeply into your cells, tissues and organs. This occurs because fluid and waste are not being picked up by the constricted lymphatic system. This can create pockets of acidic waste and fluid that will eventually become more acidic and toxic, leading to cellular malformations and tissue diseases such as cancer, polycystic diseases, lupus, candida and fibromyalgia. This imbalance into the acid side of the pH scale affects everyone in someway but we are all affected differently. ***It affects you where your circulation is limited the most.***

Your body's extensive circulatory system includes possibly millions of miles of blood and lymphatic vessels. Some vessels may be as tiny as a single strand of hair or barely visible to the naked eye. If you equate your circulation to a very intricate, and sometimes minute, plumbing system you can easily see how some tiny vessels can become congested from the constricting effects of acid and the buildup of proteins and waste.

Lymph Flow

Your blood supply is managed by a closed-loop made up of arteries and veins. The lymphatic system runs parallel to the blood system. It is another way for excess fluid and waste to return back to the heart; an "over flow mechanism." When the lymphatics are compromised you fill with fluid and cysts. Unlike the blood circulation, which is a loop, the lymphatic system is a one-way structure. It is like a river that begins around your cells with feather fine vessels called lymph capillaries, and ends in a vein before the heart. An easy way to understand the fluid circulation around your cells is to equate it to a rain forest.

I heard this explanation of how lymph flow begins in a Lymph Drainage Therapy course. Think of the trees in the rain forest as the cells in your body and the fallen leaves around the trees are spaces around your cells. As the rain falls to the ground, it begins to pool. As enough fluid builds on the surface it begins to flow following the terrain around the trees. Small pools of water merge to become small streams, which keep merging with other tributaries to become large rivers. If one tributary becomes blocked by floating wood or debris it will begin to backup. Eventually it will overflow the banks of the river, flooding the surrounding area. The river will no longer be flowing down stream but looking for alternative and inefficient routes.

This same phenomenon, a backup of fluid, happens if your lymphatic system is slowed or blocked. In the body the interstitial fluid begins to move away from the cells in pre-lymphatic pathways, which are also called tissue channels. It is similar to the rain collecting on the fallen leaves of the forest and following the terrain. The tissue channels lead the interstitial fluid from around the cells to the initial lymphatics also called lymphatic capillaries. Once the interstitial fluid enters the lymphatic capillary it is called lymphatic fluid or lymph.

Just as in plumbing when smaller drain pipes lead to larger pipes the lymph fluid flows from smaller lymph capillaries to larger pre-collectors, then to collectors and to lymph trunks or ducts. The initial lymphatics have been compared to leaky pumps. As the fluid enters the early lymph vessels, some fluid leaks out of the vessel walls, trapping and concentrating macromolecules such as proteins, lipids, carbohydrates, enzymes, urea, minerals, hormones, some dissolved gases such as carbon dioxide, cells (lymphocytes and macrophages), toxins, bacteria, metabolic waste and bits of cellular debris.

The lymphatic system can become acidic and toxic as the debris continues to enter and concentrate as it moves its way along to the thoracic duct and then to the heart. As the lymph fluid moves from vessel to vessel it may have connections to veins or pass through lymph nodes. The collecting point for most of the body's lymph is beneath the left clavicle where the thoracic duct of the lymphatic system ends in the left internal jugular vein, right before the heart.

The Lymph System's Missed Roles

To have vibrant health you must know that the lymphatic system helps to maintain the cells and tissues, recovers substances that have escaped from the blood, regulates pressure, plays an important role in immune defense, and removes fatty acids from the small intestines.

From *Silent Waves* by Dr. Chikly:

1. "The lymphatic system: Absorbs excess fluid, macromolecules (proteins), electrolytes, toxins and foreign substances (debris) from the interstitial compartments. It constantly cleanses tissue, and removes wastes, damaged and dead cells in conditions such as traumatic injuries or necrosis. Through these processes the lymphatic system helps to maintain the optimal functioning and the integrity of the connective tissue.

2. Recovers and returns to the blood circulation those substances that have escaped from the blood compartment into the tissues.

3. Regulates the fluid volume and pressure in a tissue.

4. Helps transport immunocompetent cells (lymphocytes) and other substances (i.e., hormones) throughout the body. May play an important role in the localization of infection in the body. Helps generate immunocompetent cells in the lymph nodes.

5. Carries food components (fatty acids) absorbed by the small intestines to the blood circulation."

The Lymphatic System Completes Circulation

Even though the anatomy of the lymphatic system has been studied for hundreds of years, we are only beginning to understand the workings of this vast system. It is so misunderstood that it is barely included in the ideas of disease or healing. We need to include a toxic tissue acidosis and its negative affect on the body, especially the lymphatic system, into our general knowledge of health. Many of our current medical practices and medications will have to be re-examined to see if they are enhancing or hindering lymph flow which is critical to good circulation and good health.

When you are overly acidic, excessive amounts of acidic waste and cellular debris are stored in the tissues, including your organs. As a result you become congested in one or many systems of the body. The lymphatic system is critical in completing circulation through your tissues and organs. Complete circulation through your tissues and organs is critical to optimal health. I have had more than one patient with elevated liver enzymes whose tests returned to normal after only a few sessions to activate their lymphatic system.

Look Around You for Skin Problems

Take a look around you. Notice anyone with skin problems? The next time you are in a crowd or watching the television, start taking notice of the number of people who have skin problems such as acne, skin growths, beauty marks, faded black or brown blemishes, skin growths and irregular skin tones. Why do we have so many skin problems? Your lymphatic system is responsible for keeping your skin healthy. When you are overly acidic lymph flow slows, creating excess waste, proteins, hormones and toxins in your skin that leads to impeded circulation, toxicity and cellular buildup in your skin.

As a lymphedema therapist I see skin on a daily basis. It's remarkable the amount of, so aptly named, "beauty marks", blemishes and skin growths on our skin, especially children. These beauty marks and blemishes are cellular damage. The lymph flow from these areas has been compromised. Consequently, the lymphatic system is not able to maintain that clump of cells and they become toxic and damaged.

When I map the lymphatic flow of skin problems such as acne, skin tags and beauty marks, the lymph is always flowing in the direction of the problem. At the same time the flow around the skin problem is flowing normally towards the heart. This makes it clear to me that this area is congested, which is resulting in excess cellular waste and toxins in the area of the blemish or growth. Congestion in the tissues creates small pockets of acidic waste and proteins, which over time lead to cellular damage. Your skin problems, despite how minor you may think they are, are cellular damage from over acidity and resulting toxicity.

Impeded Lymph Flow

Your health is dependant on good circulation, especially lymph flow, to keep your cells healthy. There are many circumstances that may slow or stop your lymph flow. Injury from trauma, surgery, infection, stress, negative emotions, severe cold, dehydration, bad posture, tight clothing, food additives, volatile fumes (gas and paint fumes, colognes), acidic foods and acidic beverages, all may impede circulation. Injuries don't have to be very traumatic to cause congestion in the tissues. Small bumps and bruises can damage a blood or lymph vessel and create swelling and possibly lead to inflammation and fibrosis due to limited circulation and accumulation of fibrin and other cellular debris. When a person has had many trauma's or surgeries their body becomes filled with fibrin which will limit their ability to loose weight and attain health.

CHAPTER FIVE

Important Lymphatic System Details

The lymphatic system is a very complex network of vessels and nodes that has many important parts. These details of the lymphatic system will help you better understand its importance to your health.

Superficial and Deep Lymphatic Flow

There are two levels of lymph flow, superficial (See Fig. 5.01) and deep. The superficial lymph flow is right under your skin and accounts for 60%-70% of your body's lymph. If you gently press a finger to your arm, barely touching your skin, you are interacting with the superficial lymph flow. If you press more firmly you are interacting with the deep lymphatic flow, which accounts for 30%-40% of your body's lymph. There are many factors responsible for lymph flow such as muscle contraction, contractions of adjacent arteries and external compression from manual therapies. Exercise stimulates the drainage of the skeletal muscles by 5 to 15 times. The drainage of the skin (superficial lymph flow) is not directly affected by exercise; it is mostly dependant on deep breathing and stretching of the skin.

Deep Breathing Increases Lymphatic Flow and Blood Circulation

Deep breathing is important for proper lymph flow. In his book Silent Waves, Dr. Chikly writes, "The negative intrathoracic pressure during inspiration creates a "respiratory pump" which helps to discharge lymph into the central veins. The volume of lymph that is "pumped" into the large veins depends on the depth of inspiration and the overall breathing rate."

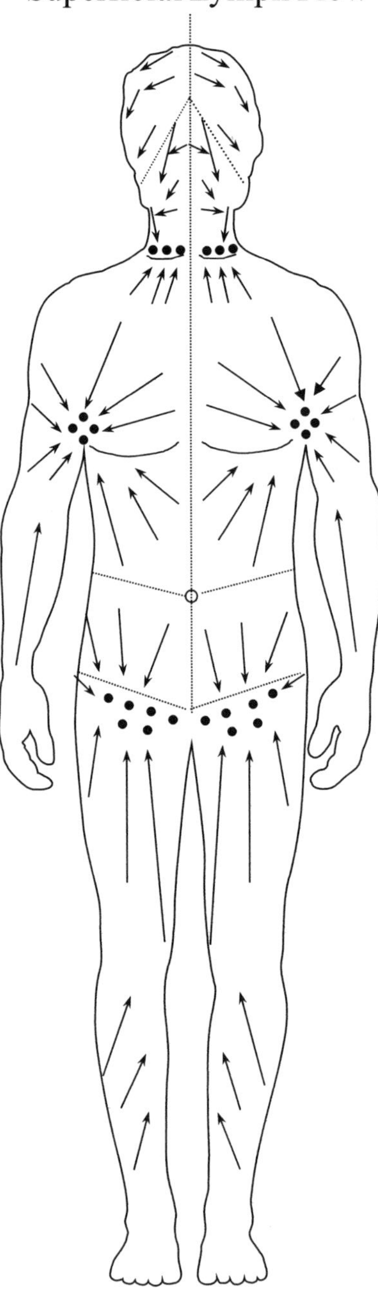

Fig. 5.01 The superficial lymph vessels drain and help maintain your skin. It's flow has a specific direction.

I have been observing people breathe for many years; we are very shallow breathers. If you are concentrating on work, you barely move your chest when you inhale. You need to breathe deeply enough to move lymph and blood through the tissues and organs. Deep breathing also pushes oxygen and nutrients deeper into your tissues and moves waste out of your tissues.

Lymph Collector
(”little hearts” of the lymph)

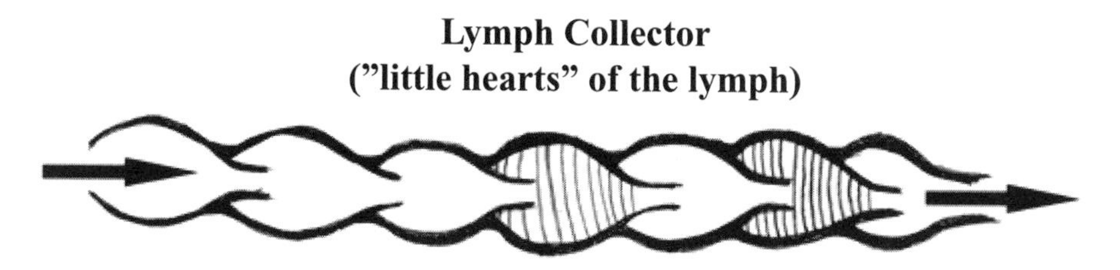

Fig. 5.02 The lymphangion of the lymph collectors consist of 2-3 layers of spiral muscular units (depicted by bands) that contract to help move lymph through the vessel.

Lymphangion or Little Hearts

Larger lymph vessels called lymph collectors have muscular units called lymphangions or “little hearts” of the lymphatic (See Fig. 5.02) When stimulated, these muscular units that form the lymph collectors, create rhythmic contractions that are critical to lymph flow. Deep breathing, exercise and lymphatic activation can stimulate the heart like muscles and increase lymph flow through the lymph vessel by some twenty to thirty times.

Cisterna Chyli

The cisterna chyli is an important group of three vessels at the beginning of the thoracic duct in your lower chest (See Fig. 5.03). It is on your right side, close to your gall bladder and diaphragm, slightly to the right of the aorta. Two of these vessels drain the lymph of your legs, the third vessel drains the intestines and pelvis. Its name comes from early researchers who observed a milky white fluid called chyle where these major lymph vessels converge. There is very rarely any actual cistern or reservoir where the three vessels converge. Chyle is lymph from your intestines produced during digestion, its white appearance comes from lipids (fats). When we look at the lymphatic system as a river, the cisterna chyli is where three rivers converge into one. This area can congest easily and create a back up of lymph in the legs, intestines and pelvis.

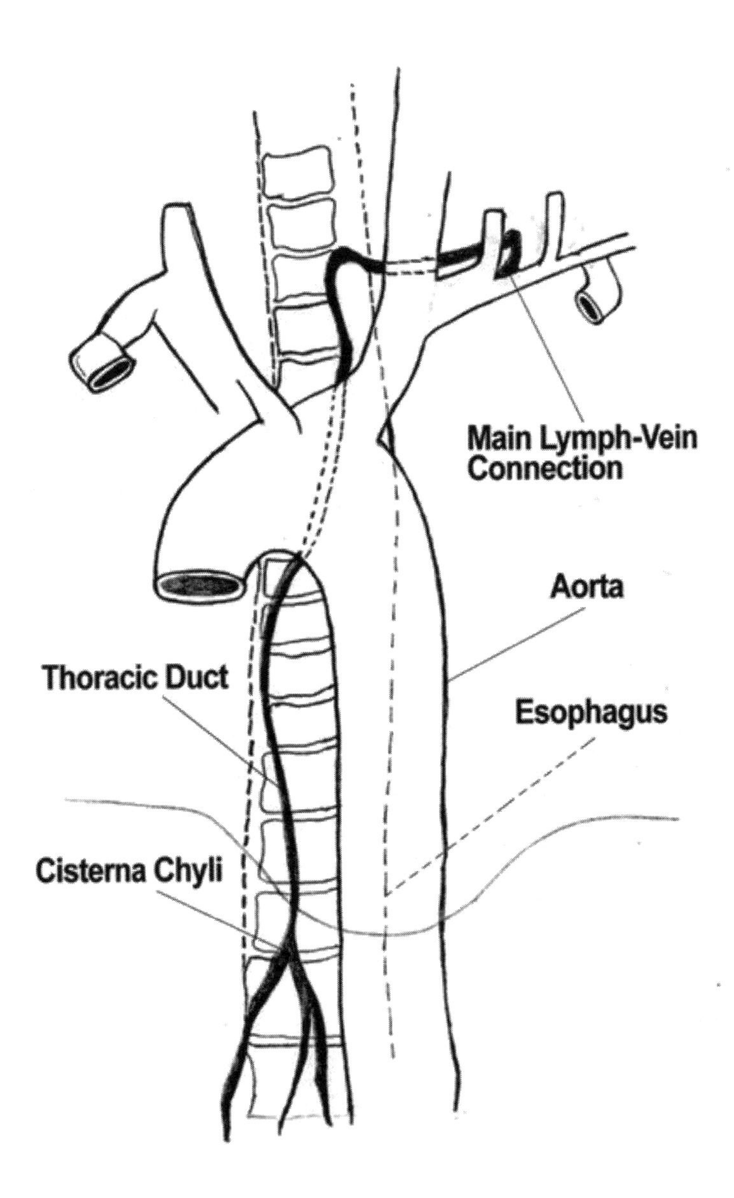

Fig. 5.03 This drawing shows the cisterna chyli, thoracic duct and main lymph-vein connection. Notice how the thoracic duct runs between the spine, aorta and esophagus. If the thoracic duct were acidic and toxic it could negatively affect the muscles of the back, spine and tissues of the esophagus or aorta.

We all drive on freeways, when three lanes converge into one there is often a slowing or back up of traffic. The same can happen with your lymphatic system. When you sit or stand in a slouched, head forward position instead of with a straight back, you may risk crimping or bending the area of the cisterna chyli. Good posture is important for efficient circulation. Remember these are bendable vessels similar to soft flexible hoses. When you slouch, the hose can kink or bend limiting circulation. This can lead to fluid problems in the abdomen, pelvis or legs, such as bloating, spider veins, varicose veins, ovarian cysts and an enlarged prostate.

Thoracic Duct

The thoracic duct is the largest lymph vessel in the body (See Fig. 5.03). It runs between the esophagus, aorta and the spine. It begins at the cisterna chyli and ends in a vein before the heart by the left clavicle. The thoracic duct collects and moves the majority of the lymph collected in the body. I believe the thoracic duct can become acidic and toxic enough, to create back spasms, erode the esophagus or cause a dangerous aortic aneurysm.

The Main Drain - Behind the Left Clavicle

In almost all cases the main lymph vessel in the body, the thoracic duct, starts in the right lower chest by your gall bladder and diaphragm. It travels up along the front of the spine to the left internal jugular vein behind the left clavicle (See Fig. 5.03). We learned that most of the lymph flow returns to the blood under the left clavicle in a vein right before the heart. This is also the dividing line where lymph flow converges.

The lymph from your face, head and neck should flow down to the base of your neck to the clavicles. Most of the lymph in the body should flow up, ending a little above the heart by the left clavicle. This is where it is important to understand how the lymph flow is similar to a river. If the river becomes congested or dammed, it stops, slows or backs up the rest of the flow. The majority of lymph flow drains to the left clavicle. Because of our tight shoulders and neck we often impede our own lymph flow to this main lymph drain.

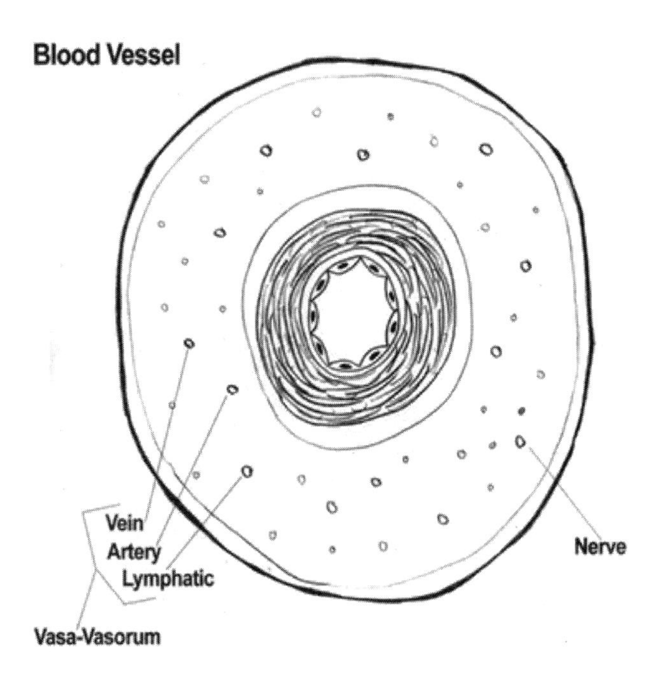

Fig. 5.04 The Vasa Vasorum are tiny blood and lymph vessels that run inside the external layer of the blood vessel to nourish the cells and clean waste.

Vasa Vasorum

Your cells depend on the circulation of nutrients, oxygen and waste. Even your blood vessels, lymph vessels and nerves are made of cells and exchange nutrients and waste with their own tiny set of nerve, blood and lymph vessels called vasa vasorum, which is Latin for "vessels of the vessels" (See Fig. 5.04).

Your blood vessels, lymph vessels and nerves each have their own distinct circulation of little vessels running inside along their length allowing for circulation that brings nutrients and removes waste.

Most of your blood vessels have three distinct layers; the exceptions are the capillaries and venules. In the outermost layer, called the Tunica Externa, you will find the vasa vasorum, a tiny set of arteries, veins, lymph vessels and nerves. I believe these tiny vessels can become backed up and become toxic from acidity and excess proteins which can cause Bell's Palsy, sciatica or a heart attack by creating a spasm in the wall of the blood vessel or nerve.

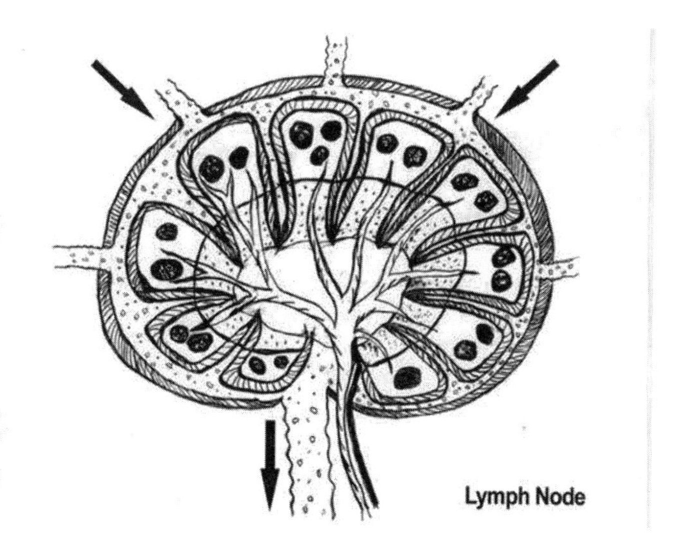

Fig. 5.05 The lymph nodes act to filter out bacteria, viruses and are very important in fighting infection and disease.

Lymph Nodes

Lymph nodes are your body's sewage treatment plants (See Fig. 5.05). There are approximately 400-700 lymph nodes in the body. Almost half of them are in the abdomen. Many more are in your neck and chest while the rest are in the creases of the body such as the underarms, crease of the upper leg, behind the knee, ankles and other areas. The wrist is the only crease that does not contain lymph nodes. A normal node can range in size from the size of a pinhead to that of a large grape.

The lymph nodes have many specific functions. When lymph flows through the nodes, immune cells such as lymphocytes destroy foreign or unwanted substances. Lymph moves out of the nodes into lymph vessels to travel to the main drain. There the waste can then easily be handled by the liver, and flushed out of the organs of elimination: the kidneys, digestive organs, skin and lungs. Lymph becomes concentrated in the nodes where about 40% of the incoming lymph is carried away by the venous system. So the lymph fluid is even more concentrated with waste and proteins as it moves through the lymph vessels and nodes towards the heart.

The nodes store large amounts of lymphocytes, which are white blood cells that fight infection and disease. The concentration of lymphocytes increases when the flow of lymph through the nodes increases. The majority of us are very sedentary, we sit at work, we sit in our cars and we sit at home.

If you are not moving your circulation by increasing your heart rate, you are not moving lymphocytes to fight infection and disease. This is a partial reason why you hear so much about needing to build your immune system. It isn't working because of a malfunctioning lymphatic system. The lymphatic system is meant to move lymphocytes, pick up waste, like toxins and help clean the tissues. Excess toxins are being concentrated in your slowed or stopped lymphatic system. This can be a reason why there are so many diseases like cancer that can involve the blood, tissues, bones, organs and lymph system.

Patient Profile: Laura T.

When Laura walked into my office, the first thing I noticed was her ashen complexion and how weak she seemed. I have learned that an ashen (deadly pale) complexion is a sign of limited circulation. When she took off her sweater, I could see a large mass protruding from the left side of her abdomen. She told me her doctor said it was an enlarged spleen. Laura has a small frame and weighs just over 100 pounds. She has also been unable to keep weight on, which was evident, she was just skin and bones. Laura had been a jewelry designer for almost twenty years. During that time she has been exposed to some very toxic chemicals. Laura's health problems began when she was in her early twenties with a severe case of chronic fatigue syndrome. She turned to manual therapies and better nutrition to help increase her energy. Laura bounced back and regained her strength. Eight years later, after another chemical exposure, she became very ill again. After many blood tests and examinations, her doctors thought she had leukemia. Laura chose again to try a macrobiotic diet and manual therapies to deal with her illness. Over time she regained her strength and her blood levels returned to normal.

A few years ago Laura decided to have her mercury filled amalgams removed from her teeth. Ensuing health problems from the dental work left her weak and ill. She turned to the macrobiotic diet again to try and build her body. It took her almost a year to regain much of her strength. No matter what she did to try to improve her health, she never felt completely well. Laura started having a problem with abscesses in her mouth right before a family cruise. This is a sign that her body was having circulation problems. Because of time constraints she decided to hold treatment off until returning from the trip. During the cruise Laura and her family went swimming with dolphins for over two-hours in extremely cold water. By that night she was extremely ill from hypothermia and went into shock. Intense cold can severely damage the lymphatic system. In less than a week she lost twenty pounds. Her health and emotional stability were rapidly declining. Laura decided to try a healthier diet again.

After months of a strict diet and massages, her health continually declined. Even though Laura was losing weight, her, legs had been filling with fluid and proteins. The lightest touch would leave a deep indentation in her legs, this is called "pitting edema." The extra weight of her swollen legs was making her less able to climb stairs or walk easily. After a few sessions of activating lymph flow in her body she was feeling more energy and her legs were feeling less full. After a series of three Lymphatic Cellular Detox Massage sessions Laura first felt very fatigued for a few days then her energy began to return. In less than three weeks Laura's friends were remarking how good her color looked. Her ashen complexion was now a healthy glow from enhanced circulation. Over two months of sporadic treatment Laura's swollen legs were reducing and she was gaining strength. Her spleen was not doing so well, it was not reducing. In one of our early sessions I explained how systemic enzymes may help to remove excess proteins from her body. After looking at the product information Laura said she wanted to see if lymphatic activation and the macrobiotic diet would work on their own.

After six weeks of seeing the therapies benefit her health, but not reduce her spleen, Laura decided to try another series of lymphatic activations. This time she also decided to try taking systemic enzymes. Two weeks later I saw Laura and her legs were doing great, barely indenting, and her spleen was much softer and a little smaller. She said it felt like it was reducing. Laura may have had a lifelong problem with her lymphatic system, evident of her many illnesses. When she went into the cold water, her already weak lymphatic system just couldn't recover and shut down from the cold water. When we manually activated her lymph flow and helped the body to remove excess proteins, fluid and acid waste she began to recover.

CHAPTER SIX

Acid + A Slowed Lymph System = Protein Proliferation

Acid can be extremely damaging. It will etch glass or marble and it will burn your skin. Internally it can negatively affect every system of your body down to the cell. Did you know you are completely made up of cells, possibly 100 trillion? The larger you are the more cells you have. Cells are made up of 90% water, 5% protein and the remaining 5% is made up of nucleic acid, lipids, carbohydrate and other substances. Your cells will group together to become all tissues in the body. These tissues become your skin, muscles, bones, organs and brain. Your ear, stomach or liver may be millions of cells that are mostly alive. To stay alive, cells must be able to carry out a variety of functions. Some cells must be able to circulate through the body while most cells must be able to divide and replicate themselves.

All cells must be able to receive oxygen, ingest nutrition and expel their waste. Cells must also be able to respond to changes in their fluid environment. For example a high acid diet, trauma, stress, dehydration, cigarettes, prescribed and recreational drugs such as alcohol and marijuana, can create changes in the cell's environment. These all negatively affect your lymphatic system's ability to clean your body and you become acidic and toxic.

If your lymphatic system is not functioning properly due to toxicity, it negatively affects your circulation which can affect every system of the body. Cellular debris including acidic waste, toxins and proteins can build in and around your cells. This buildup of cellular debris and proteins creates little log-jams, as in a river, further limiting fluid circulation to your tissues, especially your organs and brain.

Protein Proliferation

When you are injured the body repairs itself by producing fibrin, which is formed from fibrinogen, a protein found in blood. When blood vessels are damaged due to trauma, a series of reactions causes fibrinogen to coagulate (thicken) into strings of fibrin. These strings of protein proliferate and flow through the blood to the wound where they begin to lay on top of one another to form a mesh. Red blood cells, and cells called platelets, then combine with the fibrin mesh to form a clot.

Even though the body has mechanisms in place to prevent the over production of fibrin, it still gets over produced. Excess fibrin flows through your blood combining with blood cells, cholesterol, waste and cellular debris. If it attaches to damage on the blood vessel walls, as in arteriosclerosis, it can buildup and eventually create a blockage which may limit blood flow to the cells of the heart. This impeded blood flow can lead to fibrosis of the heart, heart attacks, strokes, and other life-threatening conditions. Excess fibrin can clog your lymph and blood vessels and enter your tissues and organs congesting them. Over a period of time your organs become tight and are unable to function optimally due to fibrosis and scarring.

500 Million Cells Die Daily

Approximately 500 million cells die inside your body every day. With that many cells dying each day, that small percentage of the cell that is 5% protein, can quickly accumulate as cellular debris in the blood and tissues. Cells can die in two different ways. The first way is called apoptosis, also known as "programmed cell death" in which the cell dies from its own mechanisms. This cellular death occurs often as part of the normal functioning of the human body as it rids itself of unwanted, damaged or dead cells.

The second way in which cells die is through necrosis. This may occur from an injury due to external trauma as in an accident or in surgery. Acidic internal fluids can also cause necrosis. Trauma or acid can damage tissues and blood vessels, which may impede blood supply to the cells. If cells can't receive nutrition and oxygen, or remove their waste, they become damaged and many die due to toxicity. There are many causes of necrosis besides injury such as inflammation, infection, heart attack and tissue acidosis. An easy way to distinguish between the two forms of cellular death might be to compare apoptosis to cells creating their own death and necrosis to cells having their life taken away.

Normal Life Leads To Cellular Damage and Death

Everyday millions of cells are becoming damaged and dying through the normal life process of apoptosis. If we are injured from a trauma, for example a hard bump into a table, we now have more cellular damage and death from necrosis. These damaged and dead cells can be numerous and become excess cellular debris and proteins that are floating in your blood. Now add fibrin that is rushing to create a mesh to repair damage in your body and you can easily see how you are becoming filled with cellular debris and proteins such as fibrin. This excess fibrin and cellular debris is thickening your blood. When your blood is thick it doesn't flow through your tissues and organs easily. If excess fibrin and cellular debris is not picked up from around your cells by the lymphatic system it can begin to build in your tissues and organs. This buildup is called fibrosis and leads to scarring that can limit an organ's ability to function.

Fibrosis can occur in any tissue or organ. One example is Pulmonary Fibrosis, which involves scarring of the lung. Keep in mind that the lungs help to remove acid from your body. If that ability to remove acid were impeded, your lungs would become very acidic and gradually become filled with fibrosis (protein buildup). In Pulmonary Fibrosis, the air sacs of the lungs become replaced by fibrotic tissue. As the scar forms, the lung tissue becomes thicker, causing a loss of the tissue's ability to transfer oxygen into the bloodstream. This fibrosis can also affect your heart. As the heart becomes more scarred due to fibrosis, it can lose the ability to pump blood efficiently.

Acidity Slows Our Ability to Remove Excess Proteins

In his book Alkalize or Die, Dr. Baroody writes "Lymph fluid flows best in an alkaline medium. When the body is overly acidic it slows, creating one of the most chronic, life threatening situations…"

In *Silent Waves*, Dr. Chikly writes: *"The lymphatic system: Absorbs excess fluid, macromolecules (proteins), electrolytes, toxins and foreign substances (debris) from the interstitial compartments. It constantly cleanses tissue, and removes wastes, damaged and dead cells in conditions such as traumatic injuries or necrosis. Through these processes the lymphatic system helps to maintain the optimal functioning and the integrity of the connective tissue."* The lymphatic system is critical in completing circulation through your tissues and organs. It plays an important role in removing excess proteins, waste and fluid from the body. If you are acidic, the lymphatic system's ability to remove these proteins is slowed, impeding circulation. This leads to congestion in the tissues and over time you become more fibrotic, tight, toxic and ill.

Extreme Protein Proliferation

You know that normal cell death and normal wound repair with fibrin can lead to excess protein in your blood and tissues. When you include a toxic tissue acidosis that may be damaging parts of your internal body 24 hours a day, 7 days a week, a severe fibrosis (buildup of proteins such as fibrin) can develop in your tissues. The body's repair mechanisms may be working round the clock to repair the damage from the toxic acid that is in the tissues, producing too much fibrin. When you are overly acidic your lymphatic system is not working optimally. The excess proteins are not being removed effectively from your tissues creating fibrosis and congestion in your organs. Because of an undetected tissue acidosis your tissues are being filled with extreme protein proliferation. This buildup of fibrin and cellular waste can severely affect one part of your body or systemically, throughout all tissues of the body. This buildup of waste is a major reason why many people need blood thinners as we age and why you are told to take a baby aspirin to thin your blood.

Excess Proteins in Your Urine

Excess proteins in the body are not healthy for you. Proteinuria is a condition in which there is an excess of protein in the urine. According to the Merck Manual, the major mechanism producing proteinuria is elevated blood concentrations of normal and abnormal proteins. You can test for excess proteins in the urine with specifically designed test strips. The problem occurs when you are acidic proteins can become trapped in your tissues and organs and as a result they won't be elevated in the urine. After a Lymphatic Cellular Detox Massage some patients excrete more protein than normally expected in their urine. The brochure with the test strip kit utilized to test urine protein indicated that you should not have proteins in your urine.

According to the Merck Manual, there is a specific proteinuria associated with exercising. It sometimes occurs in joggers, marathon runners and boxers who will experience high levels of proteins in their urine. When you exercise, especially intensely, you increase the deeper circulation, cleaning your body of waste and proteins. When you are sedentary, you are not moving your circulation enough to clean the waste and proteins out of your deeper tissues and you become protein filled and toxic. When I have exercised on a treadmill for 30 minutes and taken alkalizing supplements, I had high levels of protein in my urine. As I alkalize my body and move my blood by exercising, the trapped proteins can leave the tissues.

Amyloidosis – A Deadly Buildup of Cell Material

By now you should be getting the point that an overly acidic internal body constricts the lymphatic system and allows proteins to build in the tissues or organs of the body, limiting your health. In the first printing of this book I had never heard of "Amyloidosis." Fortunately while watching "House" a television show about a quirky doctor who battles to help diagnose the sick, I heard the word "Amyloidosis" when they spoke of a dying patient. I was shocked and pleased when I read the definition on MayoClinic.com "Amyloidosis is a rare and potentially fatal disease that occurs when substances called amyloid proteins build up in your organs. Amyloid is an abnormal protein usually produced by cells in your bone marrow that can be deposited in any tissue or organ. Amyloidosis can affect different organs in different people, and there are many types of amyloid. Amyloidosis frequently affects the heart, kidneys, liver, spleen, nervous system and gastrointestinal tract. The exact cause of amyloidosis is unknown,..."

The whole premise of my book is to show how the emerging science of acid-alkaline balance and the lymphatic system explains how excess proteins are slowly killing us and creating childhood diseases. So finding a disease like amyloidosis that associates abnormal proteins to many diseases and death is monumental. Some of the known symptoms of amyloidosis are swelling of your ankles and legs, weakness, fatigue, weight loss, shortness of breath, numbness or tingling, diarrhea, an enlarged tongue (macroglossia), an irregular heartbeat, difficulty swallowing, skin changes and purpura (purple discolorations around eyes) which occurs due to broken blood vessels.

Protein Buildup is a Serious Matter

There are diseases already associated with excess proteins Alzheimer's, type 2 diabetes, autism, batten disease, heart failure, fatal familial insomnia and kidney disease. Researchers are finding excess amyloid protein and neurofibrillary tangles (tau protein) in the brains of Alzheimer's patients. These tangles of cellular debris and plaque develop in neurons and surrounding areas in normal aging. In Alzheimer's disease, tau and amyloid proteins begin to overbuild in areas of the brain. Tau is a protein that helps to maintain nerve cell structure. As these proteins build in the brain they stack in layers crowding the tissue. As the layers of proteins increase, circulation through the brain tissue becomes impeded and brain function decreases. In the next chapter you will learn about an important missed lymph/brain connection, which is critical in understanding how proteins are filling the tissues of the brain creating Alzheimer's and diseases like autism. The lymphatic system is responsible for up to 48% of the drainage of cerebrospinal fluid and proteins in that fluid. A toxic tissue acidosis can create excess proteins that can build within the brain and ultimately steal the minds and lives of children and seniors.

The Overweight and Underweight are Protein Filled

If you have ever seen a picture of a cute, chubby baby with rolls of skin, you were looking at a very lymphatically challenged and congested baby. However, please don't get the idea that only individuals that have weight problems are being filled with proteins and fluid. You can be very thin and look healthy but proteins, fluid and waste may be filling your organs or bones limiting circulation. The problems may not be visible for years. Over time your body becomes more congested and unable to function optimally.

Protein Requirements

Daily protein requirements vary depending upon your size and activity level. The U.S. Government standards for protein are 0.8 gram per 2.2 pounds of body weight. An adult male who weighs 190 pounds requires approximately 70 grams of protein daily. An adult female who is 140 pounds requires about 51 grams. A large egg or small portion of beef, chicken or fish has approximately 7 grams of protein. A baked potato has 6 grams and a ½ cup of vegetables has 2-3 grams of protein. The goal is to eat more of your protein from vegetables. Besides giving you protein vegetables help to make your tissues more alkaline helping to increase lymph flow and the removal of trapped waste and proteins.

We need to re-examine the protein need in the body. We need much less protein than we think we need. Because they think they need a lot of protein in their diet many people are hurting themselves by adding whey or soy protein to their already protein filled body's.

CHAPTER SEVEN

Important Lymph Connections

Lymph/Brain Connection

If you suffer from depression, anxiety, are having problems thinking or have a child with learning disabilities, you need to understand the connection between the lymphatic system and the brain. To be more precise, the brain itself does not have any lymph vessels. The lymph/brain connection is actually a lymph/cerebrospinal fluid connection where up to 48% of cerebrospinal fluid (CSF), which bathes the brain and spinal cord, can be reabsorbed into the body via the lymphatic system. This CSF reabsorption can take place through many venues including the nasal mucosa, intracranial and extracranial nerves and parts of the meninges. The meninges are a part of the craniosacral system which runs from your head to your sacrum (base of the spine) and covers your central nervous system. Even though the craniosacral system has been researched and written about for decades, like the lymphatic system, it is not considered in diseases of the brain.

The Craniosacral System

The craniosacral system (See Fig. 7.01) is made up of structures called the meninges, choroid plexus, arachnoid villi and granulations, as well as cerebrospinal fluid. The choroid plexus is where cerebrospinal fluid is produced from your blood. The arachnoid villi and granulations are where the majority of the cerebrospinal fluid is thought to be reabsorbed back into the body. New research shows that the meninges of the craniosacral system and the lymphatic system may play an important role in cerebrospinal fluid transport and reabsorption. The meninges are membranes that surround and protect the brain and spinal cord. Have you heard of meningitis? It is a severe infection in the membranes that surround the brain and spinal cord. It can be life threatening. The meninges are made up of three layers (dura mater, arachnoid mater and pia mater) that conform to the shape of the brain and spinal cord. Two of its three layers have lymph vessels and act as a conduit to help remove cerebrospinal fluid and proteins from around the spinal cord and brain.

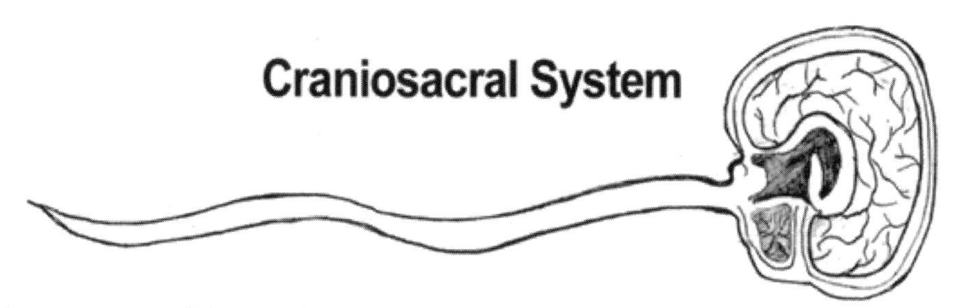

Fig. 7.01 Part of the craniosacral system, the meninges, encloses the brain and spinal cord. It has attachments in the cranium and sacrum. Separated from the body the craniosacral system would resemble a tadpole with a large head and a thin, long tail.

Lymph/Cerebrospinal Fluid Connection

The following research from Silent Waves by Dr. Chikly shows that 40–48% of cerebrospinal fluid is absorbed by extracranial lymph vessels. Extracranial lymph vessels are lymph vessels outside of the head. Many of the lymphatics that help drain the cerebrospinal fluid are located around the nasal area. If the nasal lymph vessels are slowed, CSF trying to leave the brain and enter the lymph vessels may be backing up into the sinuses or become an annoying nasal drip down the back of your throat. The studies were done on sheep because their circulation is similar to humans.

Lymph/Cerebrospinal Fluid Connection Research:

"We estimated the volumetric clearance of cerebrospinal fluid (CSF) through arachnoid villi and extracranial lymphatics in conscious sheep. We conclude that 40-48% of the total volume of CSF absorbed from the cranial compartment is removed by extracranial lymphatic vessels."

Boulton M, Flessner M, Armstrong D, Hay J, Johnston M, Determination of volumetric cerebrospinal fluid absorption into extracranial lymphatics in sheep, Am J Physiol. 1998 Jan;274(1 Pt 2):R88-96.

"There is mounting evidence that a significant portion of cerebrospinal fluid drainage is associated with transport along cranial and spinal nerves with absorption taking place into lymphatic vessels external to the central nervous system. In summary, Microfil distribution patterns in neonatal lambs illustrated the important role that cranial and spinal nerves play in linking the subarachnoid compartment with extracranial lymphatics."

Zakharov A, Papaiconomou C, Djenic J, Midha R, Johnston M, Lymphatic cerebrospinal fluid absorption pathways in neonatal sheep revealed by subarachnoid injection of Microfil, Neuropathol Appl Neurobiol. 2003 Dec;29(6):563-73.

"contrary to the established view, the Johnston study indicates that this pathway [venous system] may represent a secondary system that is recruited to compliment lymphatic transport when global absorption capacity is stressed or compromised. This *ground breaking* work could change the way we think about and treat edema of the brain, the regulation of CSF and counters the long-held belief that lymphatics do not play a significant role in the central nervous system"
Zakharov A., et al., "Integrating the Roles of Extracranial Lymphatics and Intracranial Veins in Cerebrospinal Fluid Absorption in Sheep", Microvasc. Res., 2004, Jan, 1, 67, (1): 96-104.

Toxicity = Brain Dysfunction

If you are overly acidic, your lymphatic system is slowed. The lymphatic system is responsible for almost 48% of cerebrospinal fluid absorption. If an undiagnosed tissue acidosis is slowing your lymphatic system it can create a backup of cerebrospinal fluid, acidic wastes, and proteins in the brain. This backup of debris causes congestion and may play an important role in migraines, depression, anxiety, learning disabilities, autism, Alzheimer's, and other diseases of the brain.

The Dura Mater Is Tough

The lymphatics play a significant role in maintaining the tissues of the brain, especially your dura and pia maters which contain lymph vessels. The dura mater is the top layer of the meninges and the pia mater is the layer closest to the brain and spinal cord. The dura is very fibrous and tough. I believe the dura and pia mater can become acidic enough to constrict or tighten around the spinal cord and may be a major contributing factor in back pain, neck pain, headaches, migraines, scoliosis and meningitis. When the back of your head feels like it is in a vise, or is being pulled down into your neck, it may be an acidic dura mater constricting and pulling on an area around the base of the brain or spinal cord.

Mad Cow Disease

You may be wondering why mad cow disease is in this section about the lymph/brain connection. When the first mad cow scare happened in 2003 in the United States, I had just finished rereading an article by Dr. Chikly, "Is Human Cerebrospinal Fluid Reabsorbed By Lymph?" (From The American Academy of Osteopathy (AAO) Journal 1998, 8, 2: 2834) In the article, Dr. Chikly collected a significant amount of research from many lymphatic researchers showing there are definitely many lymph/cerebrospinal fluid connections.

A representative of The National Cattlemen's Beef Association and U.S. Agriculture Secretary Ann Veneman were telling the public that the United States meat was safe because muscle cuts of meat have almost no risk of contamination. There reasoning was that the virus was contained within the brain and spinal cord area. I knew that was not true. When you include the lymph/cerebrospinal fluid connection, the mad cow virus in the brain tissue can enter the cow's muscles through the lymphatics. Research shows that up to 48% of the cerebrospinal fluid is absorbed by the lymphatics. The lymphatics clean the tissues returning the fluid, waste and possible virus back to the heart and into the blood supply to go through the organs and back into the muscles.

We all know that cows are herbivores, they are meant to eat grass. Ranchers cut costs by feeding their cows other dead cows or animals mixed with feed. This process is called rendering and is basically the grinding up of diseased, dead cows to be mixed with feed. Once you know about acid-alkaline balance and the lymph/cerebrospinal fluid connection you will see that the cows are becoming severely acidic. It is impairing their lymphatic system, which is making their brain, spinal cord and nerves toxic. The cow's symptoms include an excitable or nervous temperament when their skin is touched, (it probably hurts, acid makes the body sensitive) and an unsteady gait that results in the inability of the cow to stand up. We suffer with many of the same symptoms. Cows are meant to eat grass, they don't do well eating meat or grains because it makes them acidic, congested and toxic. Are we meant to eat as much meat as we do, and can this be adding to our toxicity and lead to diseases of the body and mind as well? YES!

Lymph/Immune System Connection

Even though we hear and read about the immune system, most individuals don't really understand what it is and how to make it stronger. In a very brief description, your immune system is made up of lymphoid organs (organs that store lymphocytes). These lymphocytes circulate through your tissues to help the body fight disease, foreign substances and play a major role in the immune response. The primary lymphoid organs are your bone marrow and thymus. Bone marrow is the spongy tissue in the center of large bones. Bone marrow contains stem cells which produce red and white blood cells. White blood cells are called leukocytes and become lymphocytes and monocytes. Monocytes that have been activated turn into macrophages that can engulf and destroy harmful microorganisms by digesting them. The thymus aids in the further development of lymphocytes. There are two kinds of lymphocytes that are formed from cells in the bone marrow. Lymphocytes called B cells, mature in the bone marrow itself. The other lymphocytes travel to the thymus where they become T cells.

The secondary lymphoid organs are the lymph nodes, spleen, tonsils, appendix, digestive tract and the lining of the respiratory tract as well as other lymphoid tissue. These lymphoid tissues contain large amounts of lymphocytes. The secondary lymphoid organs and tissues collect and store for later use, large numbers of lymphocytes that have migrated from the bone marrow and thymus. These lymph-associated tissues are where many of your health problems occur (i.e., children with autism have severe abdominal problems, many in our population have appendicitis, enlarged spleens, enlarged lymph nodes and enlarged or infected tonsils).

Circulation Improves Your Immune System

The point to be made is that in order for your immune system to function, lymphocytes and other cells that produce an immune response need to be circulating through your tissues. If you are overly acidic and toxic, your lymphatic system is constricted, limiting your circulation. This weakens your immune system by limiting the circulation of red blood cells to deliver oxygen, and white blood cells to fight infection and disease.

Recurring infections are a major problem in our country. Over acidity and limited circulation through your tissues is why many of you have recurring infections and such a weakened immune system.

Stem Cells

There is a lot of controversy over stem cells. If you weren't acidic and toxic, your cells would be healthy instead of becoming damaged and subsequently die. Stem cells are generic cells made in bone marrow, which have the ability to become any kind of cell in the body. Medical researchers believe stem cells have the potential to change the face of disease by being utilized to repair specific tissues or to grow organs. Unfortunately, they are putting healthy cells into a toxic and unhealthy environment that can damage the new healthy cells. We can increase the survival rate for stem cells by first manually increasing fluid circulation in the body, especially in the specific areas to be implanted, using lymphatic activation. This can help increase oxygen and nutrition to the new cells and help remove their waste maintaining a healthy cellular environment.

Lymph/Organ Connection

The lymphatic system has many connections throughout the entire body. There are only a few places where there are no lymph vessels, for example the sclera (the whites of the eye) and the placenta. Most places where you have blood you have lymph vessels to pick up a portion of the fluid and proteins that are left in the tissues.

Every tissue and organ has an inflow of arterial blood, an outflow of venous blood and an outflow of lymph. When the lymph is slowed, circulation through the deeper tissues of the organ can be slowed. This creates a congestion of fluid, waste and excess protein that can limit the ability of the organ to function. Fibrosis in an organ is a very common problem; it is a buildup of fibrin and other proteins. To reduce and prevent fibrosis, you need to balance your body and increase circulation in the affected organ.

CHAPTER EIGHT

Asthma, Aggression, Learning Disabled, ADHD, Asperger's and Autism

Toxicity is Hurting Children

Autism spectrum disorders are quickly becoming one of the most devastating epidemics affecting the nation's children. Many experts were hoping that in 2005 they would see an end to autism's steady rise. Unfortunately, autism rates are still climbing. In 1994, it was estimated that one in 10,000 children were autistic. In 2004 the estimate was one in 200 and in 2005 the revised estimate is that one in 166 children will be affected by autism. There is a major problem. If the exponential growth of autism persists at its present rate, estimates for 2015 are projected to be as high as 1 in 7 children being diagnosed with autism. Something is missing in our current medical model of autism that is not allowing us to see how the disease works. That missed information is tissue acidosis and its negative affect on the lymphatic system which can lead to excess acid and proteins filling structures in the brain.

Asthma is another epidemic that is affecting the young in this nation at an alarming rate. Even though it is affecting children across the nation, it is affecting minority children the hardest. In East Harlem in New York City, asthma is affecting one in four black children. Asthma attacks are due to over acidity constricting and congesting the tissues of the lungs.

If you read the newspapers or listen to the news you have seen the enormous problem of extreme aggression and killing from children and teens. These kids are toxic and its affecting how they think. It doesn't have to be that serious to be a problem, if your child has a constant runny nose and cold they are overly acidic and toxic. All these problems may have a common denominator, tissue acidosis and its toxic affect on the lymphatic system and brain.

A Revelation / Acid Sours Breast Milk

When I first found out about an acidic pH, I had this revelation that allowed me to see how a toxic acidosis is affecting infants. I had stopped by to see my daughter's first dance class when she was four years old. In the waiting room there was a mother with her eight-month-old daughter. In our conversation she mentioned that her baby was throwing up, had stomach pains and was on two acid medications. This is an eight-month-old child. Before I mentioned anything about pH, the mother told me that her breast milk at times would taste sour or bad. At that moment I realized how this undetected tissue acidosis was affecting newborns. When the mom tested her saliva pH she was severely acidic at 5.1, her acidic body was souring the breast milk and making the baby acidic and sick. This is one reason for the prevalence of colic and acid problems affecting so many newborns.

I have seen this acidity in newborns many times in the past, even infants that are two weeks old are placed on acid medications. A good place to start looking at this problem would be in a pediatrician's office. I wonder what percentage of newborns to one year olds, are on antacids? These children are starting life with a sour stomach from mom's sour breast milk or protein laden formula. Over time their gastrointestinal tissues become more acidic which slows their lymphatic system, more specifically the cisterna chyli (three vessels by right rib cage) leading to congestion in the abdomen and body. Look around, many infants have round distended abdomens and chubby legs.

This stagnant, acidic and protein filled fluid can lead to earaches, excess fluid in the ear and infections that are affecting infants in great numbers. I believe a toxic tissue acidosis, and its negative effect on the lymphatic system, is the missing link to the increase in colic, recurring colds and infections, infant cancer, epidemic levels of asthma, aggression, learning disabilities, ADD/ ADHD, Asperger's and autism. Breastfeeding is extremely important for your infant, breast milk has antibodies to help protect the infant from bacteria and viruses. It is a complete form of nutrition, that is easy to digest compared to formula. Recent studies have shown that babies who are not breast fed for 6 months are more likely to develop a wide range of infectious diseases including ear infections, diarrhea, respiratory illnesses and have more hospitalizations. Breast feeding is very important try it for as long as you can possibly do it.

Toxic and Congested Children

Children are being harmed severely by this undetected tissue acidosis. Over the years I have seen children with tight muscles, headaches, migraines, hydro cephalus, ADHD, Tourette's, Asperger's and autism. Since learning about acidosis and its affect on the lymphatic system, I can now see that these children were severely acidic, which made them tight, congested and toxic. After a few sessions of combined CranioSacral Therapy and Lymph Drainage Therapy to improve circulation most children are more relaxed and have fewer symptoms. Children who are hyperactive become calmer, recurring infections stop and those who have problems concentrating, start to think clearer.

There's no mystery as to why these children feel better, improved circulation that improves balance in the body and brain. With improved circulation, acidic wastes, toxins and proteins that have been making these children toxic can move out of the tissues and brain into the lymphatic system, through the lymph nodes and organs, to be cleaned and eliminated from the body. By increasing the circulation of lymph and blood through the tissues, the cellular environment becomes less acidic and healthier. The children's digestive tissues and muscles begin to relax as circulation increases.

Three Short Profiles of Children

I have worked with many children with different degrees of cognitive problems for over thirteen years. Even though I often saw improvement while working with these children, the results have been more dramatic since learning about acid-alkaline balance and its affect on the lymphatics and brain. Each of the three following children went through a series of Lymphatic Cellular Detox Massage sessions to increase lymph flow and cerebrospinal fluid circulation. Two of the three children had remarkable results after the manual detoxification.

One six-year old girl who was on a diet to restrict gluten and casein, still had difficulties with her digestion, muscle tightness, hand-eye fixations, often repeating the same sentences and being emotionless (rarely smiled). After one of our first series of sessions of activating her lymphatic and craniosacral systems, the little girl jumped off my therapy table, put on her shoes and then tied them within 15 seconds. Her mother looked at me and said in a shocked voice, "that normally takes her fifteen minutes." The next session when I saw the girl she was more relaxed, less tight, animated, smiling and her mother said she was repeating herself less. After a series of sessions and seeing positive improvements, their sessions became less frequent. The benefits gained through therapy regressed slightly. I had just learned of acid-alkaline balance and didn't understand its true importance in problems of the mind. These were the first parents I showed how to manually drain their daughter using a specific routine. I was amazed at how quickly the parents were able to learn the routine and do it well.

This next young boy with autism is almost a teenager. He has survived lymphoma as child, has a problem with hitting others, speaks limited sentences and needs to be moving all the time. When I am treating him he is only on the table for a few minutes at a time until he has to get up and move about the room, then he will get back on the table. If he wants to sit in a chair, I treat him in the chair until I can coax him back onto the table. His muscles were very tight, especially his low back. When touched his skin it would turn red or get hives, a sign of toxicity in the superficial lymphatic system. I was fortunate to be able to treat this child on two different occasions during the year for a series of lymphatic activations.

The first sessions consisted of 30–40 minutes, one week apart. I used a combination of CranioSacral Therapy and Lymph Drainage Therapy over six weeks. Even though his tight body relaxed, his mother saw no improvement in her son after the sessions. Six months later I asked them to try a more specific routine I had developed. The child had a 30–40 minute Lymphatic Cellular Detox Massage session on three days close together and then twice a week for the next two weeks. Besides seeing his muscles relax again, especially those in his low back, his mother said she saw no cognitive improvement. I understand why some patients get good results and others don't. It all depends on how toxic and congested they are. This child had lymphoma, so he already had a compromised lymphatic system to start with; his tight muscles verify the acidity in his tissues. When children are very toxic and congested they need more than just lymphatic activation and a few basic supplements. Following an 80/20 diet, hydration, alkalizing products, systemic enzymes and lymphatic activation are important steps in helping to decongest a child's deeper circulation of the brain.

My son, who had just turned five, had experienced small health problems since birth. When he was an infant he was a chubby baby and his body would become tight and stiff. On one of our visits to the doctor, when he was one years old, we were told that his head was large for his age group. The doctor didn't seem to be too concerned when he told us, so we didn't worry about it. My son also appeared to be extremely bloated. I didn't know it at the time but he was very acidic and congested, which was allowing fluid to retain in his body and head. If your doctor tells you that your child's head is large, there may be a problem. Take immediate action to check you child's pH, then find a licensed therapist who can increase your child's lymph flow and craniosacral circulation.

With massage and other manual therapies to improve lymphatic flow my son's body began to relax and he lost weight quickly. As he turned two, he had severe constipation and a few spots of eczema that would actually bleed occasionally no matter how hard I worked on them. He began having severe meltdowns where he would become uncontrollable and aggressive. As he became older he had a problem with aggression when things didn't go his way. He would act out and hit his older sister or us, when something upset him. There were times he would zone out for periods of time or growl at me when he was mad. The worst was when he would totally ignore me for hours, as if I weren't in the room with him. He would also be in the time out chair ten times a day. When we learned about acid-alkaline balance we gave him an alkalizing product called SeaAloe. His skin problems and constipation were gone within a few weeks, he also seemed more calm.

I have always treated my son with massage, CranioSacral Therapy and Lymph Drainage Therapy. I believe it is what may have kept him from having more severe cognitive problems. When I finally put my son through a series of Lymphatic Cellular Detox Massage sessions the results were remarkable. The first night he had a minor healing crisis where his problems worsened for a few hours. The night after the second lymphatic activation he was bouncing off the walls crying for hours, nothing would console him. My wife and I actually both cried holding him because we felt so helpless. He finally exhausted himself and fell a sleep. By the third session he was a totally different child. My wife and I were shocked to see how good he was behaving, no hitting, no growling and he was more affectionate. This only lasted two days and then he was a terror again. The detox had opened his circulation and he was doing better. As he became congested and toxic again his problems returned but not as severe.

We started giving him one systemic enzyme per day and the next week we did another series of Lymphatic Cellular Detox Massage sessions. This time he was just a little grumpy for part of an afternoon and there was no intense healing crisis, but he immediately started behaving and thinking better. Knowing how to open the lymph/brain connection saved my son, he is a normal hyperactive five year-old. I can tell when my son is becoming more toxic, some minor behavioral problems begin to return. When I notice this, I try to balance his body and activate his lymphatics for 15 minutes a few nights in a row. Sometimes he needs to be cleaned deeper with longer sessions. In between longer sessions, I give him a quick two to five-minute session to activate his lymphatics. It makes an immediate difference. Manual maintenance with CranioSacral Therapy and Lymph Drainage Therapy, even done at home by the parents, is helpful in keeping cognitive problems under control.

Manual Maintenance or Problems Return

The positive results gained from lymphatic activation will recede some as the body becomes toxic and congested again. As they continue eating excessive amounts of acidic food as well as medications, inactivity and dehydration, some of the problems gradually return. Manual maintenance is an essential key to keeping children open and thinking clearly. Professional bimonthly or monthly manual maintenance to open the body and enhance the lymph flow will help keep children flowing and functioning with fewer symptoms. Parents can learn the 2-minute manual routine in the back of this book to keep the child flowing and less toxic between sessions. My children were 5 and 7 when they learned the Two-Minute Routine to activate their lymphatics. The combination of lymphatic activation, alkalizing products and especially systemic enzymes, are important steps in ridding the body and brain of protein buildup and congestion.

Gluten and Casein Free - Only the Tip of the Iceberg

Many parents of autistic children are aware of the Gluten Free and Casein Free Diet. Studies have shown that certain foods such as gluten (the protein in wheat, oats, rye & barley) and casein (the protein in milk products), may affect neurological processes in some children, causing autistic behavior. There is research that suggests that foods containing gluten and casein should be avoided by autistic children. Some parents who restrict gluten and casein from their child's diet have told me they see improvements in behavior and cognitive function while on the diet. These children may have normal pH tests due to acid wastes storing in the tissues and not making it out into the urine. Even though the restricted diet may have cleansed the body slightly, especially the blood and initial tissues, it is still not enough to liberate the acidic waste, proteins and toxins that are stuck in the deeper tissues, including the organs and brain.

The Next Step, Try Reducing Acid

I believe moving towards a more alkalizing diet by removing more of the acid forming foods and beverages is also an important step in helping children, especially those with cognitive problems. It doesn't make sense to go through a detoxification or take expensive supplements to increase circulation when the child is eating a high acid diet that may limit circulation. Going through a series of Lymphatic Cellular Detox Massage sessions or bodywork such as CranioSacral

Therapy and Lymph Drainage Therapy are necessary for opening the deeper circulation in these children. As with any healing crisis, these children will have a regression in cognitive function and a worsening of all traits specific to that child during a lymphatic activation. The healing crisis should last a few hours to a day or two. The improved circulation is overloading the body with more acidic waste and proteins. Some children should go through lymphatic activation slowly, in shorter periods, to avoid a healing crisis. When the child is less toxic they will be able to better tolerate a series of Lymphatic Cellular Detox Massage sessions.

Hydrocephalus, Learning Disabled, ADHD, Asperger's and Autism

The above diseases affect the brain and cognitive function of millions of children. In all cases the Merck Manual and leading experts say they don't understand the cause. When we include that these children may have been acidic, toxic, and that their lymphatic systems were compromised, new light will be shed on these diseases. More importantly, prevention of these diseases and a possible cure can be found. The research we have previously seen from 1998, 2003 and 2004 indicates that 40–48% of cerebrospinal fluid (CSF), the fluid that surrounds your brain and spinal cord, is absorbed by the lymphatic system. I believe this missed information is extremely important and adds new insight into the disease process of the brain.

Our current medical model of cerebrospinal fluid reabsorption (how the fluid that surrounds the brain is reabsorbed into the body), says that structures around the brain called arachnoid villi and granulations, reabsorb the majority of the CSF. As I previously mentioned, this new research shows that 40-48% of the CSF is absorbed by the lymphatic system. This is a tremendous missed lymph/brain connection. When you are toxic your lymphatic system is compromised, impeding circulation in the body, including the brain, spinal cord and nerves. My pH studies indicate that between 43-51% of those tested are severely acidic. This over acidity leads to a malfunctioning lymphatic system, which can cause a dangerous buildup of toxins, acidic waste and proteins in the CSF and brain. Congestion can lead to enlarged or under developed structures in the brain by limiting circulation into or out of an organ. I believe this buildup of waste and proteins has a devastating affect on the brain function of children. Many parents of autistic children say they watched their child regress over time. The child could have been completely normal and then at about the age of 15 months the parents began to notice changes. If the child was previously speaking, many parents watched as their child slowly lost the ability to make sentences or to speak. I believe that in children with aggression, learning disabilities, ADHD, Asperger's and autism, the tissues, organs and structures of the brain are slowly becoming acidic, protein filled and congested. At some point the organs and brain may become partially congested or more severely congested and shut down, and the child becomes more dysfunctional or looses the ability to think clearly.

It's important to understand that with autism and hydrocephalus both have enlarged ventricles in common. The ventricles house the choroid plexus, which produce the majority of cerebrospinal fluid (CSF) from the blood. Enlargement of the ventricles can occur when CSF production exceeds reabsorption. If fluid flow is impeded in an organ, it can become enlarged or underdeveloped. Once we realize that being overly acidic slows lymph flow, the research showing that 40-48% of CSF is absorbed by lymphatic system becomes very significant in understanding diseases of the brain, like autism and hydrocephalus. Many diseases of the brain are circulation problems.

According to the Merck Manual, CT scans have isolated a subgroup of autistic children with enlarged ventricles, and MRI has recently identified a subgroup of autistic adults with hypoplasia (underdevelopment) of the cerebella vermis. Also according to the Merck Manual, "Hydrocephalus, ventricular enlargement with excessive CSF, is the most common cause of abnormally large heads in newborns. It occurs when CSF production exceeds reabsorption; ..." We are missing the lymphatic systems role in completing circulation and reabsorbing excess fluid, even in the brain.

Vaccinations

Some children start life with an undetected acidic pH that slows the lymphatic system. This may lead to fluid congestion in the head and lungs, as well as ear infections and rashes. It may also lead to repeated antibiotic use for infections. Children are then given inoculations starting at two months old and continuing for the next two years. Vaccinations are bad for our body, and not just because of mercury, a dangerous heavy metal which was used in the preparation of many vaccinations. Mercury is a neurotoxin that in low levels in the body has been shown to affect intelligence.

A vaccine is a foreign substance put into the body that creates an immune response and inflammation. If your lymphatic system was functioning optimally the problems of mercury in the tissues, and inflammation associated with vaccines, wouldn't be as serious. Your lymphatic system, when functioning optimally, helps to remove mercury and other harmful affects from the vaccines. To your body, the vaccine is an invasion of your cells. The body's defense mechanism is to produce more white blood cells, which try to overcome the invading pathogens. This creates inflammation and cell death that further impedes your malfunctioning lymphatic system and can create a buildup of waste and proteins in the tissues and brain. Over time the inflammatory affects of repeated vaccines and excess cellular waste may be causing congestion and diminished cognitive function in children. Many parents of autistic children told me that after their first vaccination their child was on multiple rounds of antibiotics for infections, sometimes for months.

Antibiotics and Congestion

The word antibiotic means against life. Anti = against, and biotic = life. Antibiotics can create a great deal of cellular damage and cellular death. This can create excess cellular debris in the blood and tissues, further limiting circulation in an already congested body. A study published in February 2004 in the journal of the American Medical Association suggests that there may be a link between the use of antibiotics and breast cancer, the second leading cause of death among American women.

Researchers reviewed medical information on 10,000 women in the state of Washington. They compared a group with breast cancer and a group without the disease. They found that women with increased antibiotic use appeared to have a greater risk of breast cancer. Antibiotics lead to excessive cellular death which may be creating congestion in these women. This congestion may lead to limited circulation in their tissues, beginning the disease process.

Can inflammation from vaccinations and excessive antibiotic use be congesting children? Once you understand the lymphatic system and the lymph/brain connection, the answer is yes. To help alleviate the congestion and problems associated with vaccinations or antibiotic use bring your child for lymphatic activation to help detox the buildup of cellular waste from the tissues of the body after vaccinations or antibiotic use.

Watch How Your Children Eat, Drink and Play

You only need to look at what your children are eating or drinking to see that they may be acidic. Their diet is almost entirely acid. They eat white bread, pancakes, frozen waffles, eggs, chicken, spaghetti, hamburgers, macaroni and cheese, pizza, chocolates, candy and drink large amounts of soda or juice from concentrate. These are all acid forming in the body. Acidic diets can affect the minds of your children by limiting circulation in their central nervous system. Help your to child think clearer by greening their diet, making sure they are drinking enough water and lymphatic activation. One of the biggest problems is making sure your child is well hydrated, monitor their water intake.

I'm encouraged to see that many schools are removing the candy and soda machines from their campuses. Schools that do not remove candy and soda machines or fill them with healthier alternatives are less interested in the welfare of their students than in the profits from the sales of such products. In the newspapers you have read how some schools are beginning to choose healthier alternatives like 100% fruit juice instead of soda. Beware of what constitutes a healthy alternative, fruit juice from concentrate is too sweet. A better alternative would be natural organic apple juice. How about having water bottles in the soda machines. Most school lunches offer various choices such as pizza, burgers, grilled cheese, and macaroni and cheese. Unfortunately, most of these are acid forming, which may be adding to your child's hyperactivity and other health problems. The next step would be for the school dietician to learn about acid-alkaline balance and make small changes to adjust the school lunches to help balance your children and help them to think clearer.

Coffee Is Not Cool

Your teenagers are very impressionable and they want to be cool. Coffee beverages have become the new cool drink for teens. What's more grown up than sitting in a coffee shop with your friends drinking sugary, sweet coffee concoctions? Even ice cream shops now offer coffee drinks. Coffee is extremely acid forming and can make teens very toxic, adding to their already tumultuous emotional states.

Computer Games Are Stressful

Stress is a known contributing factor in most diseases. It's not only our diet that affects pH, stress, inactivity and dehydration are all a big part of the equation. Remember stress is very acid forming. Children who sit for hours in front of a computer, on games such as racing, playing sports or shooting aliens are being stressed. Computer games may not seem like a great deal of stress, but a little bit of stress for extended periods of time is unhealthy. Besides the stress, if your child is in front of the computer they aren't out moving their blood.

When I was a child we weren't allowed to watch television all day long and computers weren't around, so we were outside playing. It's important for your children to get exercise because it helps to circulate their blood and clean their systems of acidic waste, proteins and toxins. Many children are too sedentary, which will affect them their whole life. When I realized that circulation is critical to my children's health I started ensuring that they get some type of exercise almost daily. We go to the park, kick a ball around, throw a Frisbee, ride bikes, jump on a rebounder (a mini trampoline) or walk on a treadmill. Once and a while I take my kids to the park and we run a few sprints to really open their circulation. A jump rope is an inexpensive way to get children to exercise.

Children are Killing Themselves and Each Other

Children are very aggressive towards each other, they are even killing each other. I was amazed at the first form my wife had to fill out for our daughter to go to kindergarten. The questionnaire listed questions such as "How aggressive is your child? Do they hit other children?" You have heard or read in the news about youths taking the lives of other children or bringing weapons to school. It's as if they have absolutely no regard for others. I have seen this same trait of acting out with aggression, with no regard to the feelings of the person they are hitting or hurting, in children with ADHD, Asperger's Syndrome (a milder form of autism) and in those with autism. I believe aggression is a form of the autism spectrum disorder. We have many labels for our children's problems, but it really comes down to how toxic and protein filled are they.

Many of my patients who have gone through a series of sessions to activate their lymphatics, remarked that as their acidity rose, they experienced restlessness, aggression, anxiety, and depression and were unable to focus their mind clearly. Doesn't this seem like ADD or autism? I believe over acidity and a slowed lymphatic system are a contributing factor as to why teens and young adults are committing suicide. Keep in mind the large missed lymph/brain connection. When they are overly acidic it clogs the lymphatic system, which affects the cerebrospinal fluid surrounding their brain and spinal cord. When their brain is not performing optimally due to acidity and lymph congestion, they think differently.

According to The American Academy of Child and Adolescent Psychiatry, in recent years, suicides among young people have dramatically increased nationwide. Each year in the U.S., hundreds of thousands attempt suicide and thousands of teenagers commit suicide. These children are toxic and not thinking clearly.

Black Box Warning

At the end of 2004, the Food and Drug Administration (FDA) asked manufacturers of many antidepressant drugs to include in their labeling a Black Box Warning. This is a very serious type of warning. They are warning you to watch for adverse affects while using the medication. In the statement they recommend close observation of adult and pediatric patients treated with antidepressants for worsening depression or the emergence of suicidal thinking and behavior. In 2005 the FDA told the maker of Strattera, a drug used for attention deficit disorder, to alert physicians and include a Black Box Warning on their product. The warning states that children being treated with Strattera should be closely watched for a worsening of their symptoms, unusual changes in behavior, as well as irritability, suicidal thoughts or actions. This worsening occurred during the beginning of therapy or when the dose was changed. Sales of Straterra were $243 million in the first six months of 2005. The FDA estimates doctors wrote a record number of antidepressant prescriptions for children (about 11 million) in 2002. The FDA also estimates that sales of antidepressant drugs in the U.S. increased from 14 million prescriptions in 1992 to 157 million in 2002. There is obviously a major problem. It would seem that as sales of prescription antidepressants increased, so did teen suicide rates. I have a suspicion that many of our medications are acid forming and interfere with lymph flow, which can interfere with the way we feel and think.

Suggestions for Children

The importance of understanding acid-alkaline balance and the lymphatic systems roles in helping to maintain the health of your children cannot be overstated. Keeping your kids hydrated will be your best defense. They should be drinking water and some natural or organic alkalizing fruit juices, not from concentrate. If your child drinks juice from concentrate try blueberry or pomegranate juice and use it to flavor their water instead as a beverage by itself.

Start greening their diet. Have more fruits and vegetables with meals. Don't torture them in order to get them to eat vegetables. Try to make it fun by including the children in the food preparation and adding vegetables they like to eat. Slowly switch almond butter (alkaline) for peanut butter (acid). Follow the steps in this book and change some of their current snacks for healthier snacks. Learn how to properly use nutritional supplements that alkalize, and systemic enzymes that help remove proteins from their body and brain. If your child has health and cognitive problems, then improving their circulation is key in balancing tissue pH and in cleaning proteins from the tissues. Lymphatic activation therapies such as CranioSacral Therapy, Lymph Drainage Therapy and Lymphatic Cellular Detox Massage are essential to creating circulation in the deeper parts of the organs like the brain.

Teach Kids Early

When you aren't watching your diet closely, you may develop gas. When someone passes wind or has flatulence, my children who were 5 and 6 would snicker and say; "someone's out of balance" and then say "they need to eat more vegetables!" I think this is tremendous and it shows our children can learn health basics at an early age. It took me 45 years to learn that having gas (a life-long problem) meant my digestion was out of balance. I thought having gas and being bloated was a normal part of life. Educating your children on acid-alkaline balance and the lymphatic system should start as early as possible.

10 Things to Teach Your Children

1. To drink enough water at one time to wet their organs not just their mouth. Drink big gulps often and not wait until they are thirsty.
2. Explain how deep breathing two times in a row helps to move waste from their body.
3. To check their urine, if it is cloudy or dark they may need more water.
4. To check their stool, if it is shaped like a log it is healthy, if it is small tight balls they are constipated and may be dehydrated.
5. What foods are alkaline and healthy and what foods are acid and not healthy.
6. Explain why they need daily exercise to move their blood to clean their body of waste.
7. Make exercise fun and do it with them.
8. To take five minutes a day to sit quietly, deep breathe and relax their mind and body.
9. How comforting a hug can be.
10. How to self-activate their lymphatic system.

CHAPTER NINE

It May Begin in the Womb

I believe this undetected tissue acidosis is causing problems for children, starting in the mother's womb. You have learned that an overly acidic internal environment is very caustic to your lymphatic system, tissues and organs of the body. What happens when the developing embryo, and then fetus, is in the mother for nine months and mom is unknowingly severely acidic? Is there complete protection for the baby inside the amniotic sac? Knowing about tissue acidosis and the lymphatic system, I don't feel there really is that complete protection that we often hear about. I have been studying the craniosacral system (membranes that support and house the brain and spinal cord) since 1995. All information regarding cerebrospinal fluid (CSF) illustrates that structures in the brain, called arachnoid villi and granulations, absorb the majority of CSF. In Chapter Seven we looked at new research that indicated 40-48% of the cerebrospinal fluid is absorbed by the lymphatics. *The following research further explains how the fetus is mostly dependent on the lymphatic system for CSF absorption until birth, when arachnoid villi and granulations begin to appear.*

This new research is critical in understanding autism and other mental disorders affecting many children in epidemic proportions. The research shows the brain of the fetus is dependent on its lymphatic system to help remove cellular waste and proteins until birth. If the lymphatic system of the fetus is compromised, the brain can become filled with cellular waste, proteins and fluids. This is how diseases of the mind begin whether they affect children who became congested in the womb or as they become teens and adults and continue to congest as waste and proteins build in their brain. This buildup of waste that can begin in the womb is a leading factor in autism spectrum disorders, depression, anxiety and bipolar disorder.

Neonatal Research

"Arachnoid villi and granulations are thought to represent the primary sites where cerebrospinal fluid (CSF) is absorbed. However, these structures do not appear to exist in the fetus but begin to develop around the time of birth and increase in number with age. ...CSF transport occurred through multiple lymphatic pathways. An especially important route was transport through the cribriform plate into extracranial lymphatics located in the nasal submucosa. These data demonstrate an essential function for lymphatics in neonatal CSF transport and imply that arachnoid projections may play a limited role earlier in development."

Papaiconomou C., Bozanovic-Sosic R., Zakharov A., Johnston M., "Does Neonatal Cerebrospinal Fluid Absorption Occur via Arachnoid Projections or Extracranial Lymphatics?", Am J Physiol Regul Integr Comp Physiol, 2002, Oct; 283, (4): R869-76.

Is the Fetus Protected?

Understanding the lymphatic system and its role in circulating blood through the tissues, I can still only speculate as to whether a mother's acidic internal environment will negatively affect her unborn child. The placenta is believed to help protect the fetus and filter the mother's blood before entering the umbilical cord. The placenta evolves after conception from the mother's own tissues and does not contain lymph vessels. If the mother's tissues were to be unknowingly overly acidic, in my opinion the placenta could also be slightly or severely acidic and become constricted. The placenta can easily become protein filled and toxic if the mother is unknowingly overly acidic and consuming too much protein. Alerting obstetricians to watch for tissue acidosis by testing saliva and urine pH, and educating expecting parents about this information, may help prevent autism and many of the diseases that are affecting infants in great numbers.

Mom and Fetus are Filling with Proteins

Preeclampsia in pregnancy is a toxic buildup of waste and proteins from the mother and the baby, overloading the mother and fetal system. Preeclampsia used to be referred to as toxemia of pregnancy, it is a toxic reaction. The mother will often have hypertension, swelling, excess protein in her urine and feel horrible. This is due to being acidic and protein filled, which impairs the lymphatic systems ability to clean your tissues. Often the patient is prescribed bed rest and increased fluids. What pregnant mothers really need to do is slowly clean their systems by eating a greener diet, drinking more mineralized water, deep breathing and doing very light exercise to move their blood and lymph in order to SLOWLY clean their toxicity. A massage, specific detox therapy or intense exercising will be too much for someone with preeclampsia. A short (30 minute) CranioSacral Therapy session is a very gentle and effective way to slowly increase circulation to help gently detox the mom and fetus during pregnancy, especially during the first trimester.

Batten Disease – Congested Children

Batten disease is a rare, fatal, inherited neurodegenerative disorder that begins in childhood. It is associated with excess proteins and fat that builds in the brain of infants (Jansky-Bielschowsky) and juveniles (Batten disease). These diseases are associated with an abnormal pigment, called lipofuscin, accumulating in the brain. Lipofuscin is a brownish pigment that remains after the breakdown and absorption of damaged cells. The brown spots on your arms that we call age or liver spots; are a buildup of lipofuscin, dead cell material. Remember you become congested and protein filled where your circulation is most impeded. There is evidence that shows that in these diseases the brain cells are having problems with removing and recycling proteins in the brain. These disorders can lead to gait problems, seizures, blindness, inability to think clearly, mental retardation, and early death. Acidosis and a malfunctioning lymphatic system can lead to excess proteins and accumulating cellular debris in the brain. In Batten disease balancing the body, systemic enzymes and lymphatic activation are key to helping these children.

Still Looking in the Wrong Place

In testing the pH of newborns, we utilize the umbilical artery. By testing the blood for pH we are again missing the fact that blood is cleaner than your tissues and we consist primarily of tissues. Saliva and urine testing is a better indicator of tissue pH. We should be testing saliva and urine to see whether acid is being released from the tissues or being stored due to acidity and congestion in the tissues. I attempted to contact various autism and OB/GYN doctors to get answers to some of my questions, but they did not return my letters or telephone calls. Even the Autism researchers who I actually met with disregarded my information. They didn't understand acidosis and the lymphatic system. Remember this doesn't fit into their medical model. I am left to speculate in the hope of opening the mind of at least one doctor or researcher who will see the severity of this information and take action. Even though I say speculate, I have collected pH data from new mothers as well as pregnant women and found that they were overly acidic.

Newborns with Health Problems

It is important to understand that many children are born with health problems such as asthma, muscular dystrophy, polycystic kidney disease, cystic fibrosis of the lungs, hydrocephalus, blindness and auto immune diseases. I believe this undetected tissue acidosis and its affect on the lymphatic system in the pregnant mother is why children are being born with these serious diseases. We already understand that acidosis and its negative affect on your circulation is a major contributing factor in disease. What could have affected a newborn to cause these same diseases? Genetics may play a role, but I believe it begins with a combination of overly acidic amniotic fluid, overly acidic fetal tissues and higher than normal protein levels in the blood and tissues of the mom and fetus.

The lungs of a fetus are not fully developed until the last few weeks prior to birth. While the lungs are developing, the fetus is moving amniotic fluid in and out of its mouth and organs. The amniotic fluid is produced by the inner lining of the sac (amnion) as well as a contribution of fluid from the baby's lungs and kidneys (metabolic waste). The amniotic fluid helps to protect, cushion and also plays an important part in developing many of the baby's vital internal organs like the lungs, kidneys, and intestines. The fetus is continually swallowing the amniotic fluid during the pregnancy. Remember the lungs and kidneys remove acid from the body, so they are adding waste to the amniotic fluid. I believe the amniotic fluid can be protein filled, acidic and not as clean and nourishing as it should be due to over acidity and a slowed lymphatic system in the mother and baby.

Since the baby is in the amniotic fluid for nine months, the fluid only has to be slightly more acidic and protein filled than normal to slowly harm the baby by allowing proteins to build in the tissues of the body and brain. This weak acidity and excess proteins can, over time, lead to a malfunctioning lymphatic system which limits circulation. This can negatively affect the lungs, limbs, organs or brain and can be a contributing factor to the epidemic levels of asthma, ADHD, autism and other diseases that are hurting children.

Looking Outside the Box

The medical community is not willing to look outside their existing medical box. It must fit into their current medical paradigm in order for them to accept anything. I have heard this from doctors time and time again. One doctor actually reprimanded me for writing about autism and Alzheimer's in the same letter. Both of these diseases are associated with excess protein in the brain. If we don't look outside of the box, how will we find new answers? I believe that is why a cure for many of our current diseases such as autism, cancer, diabetes and multiple sclerosis has not been found. We haven't looked at the true cause, a toxic tissue acidosis and its negative affect on the lymphatic system.

According to medical references, the amniotic fluid's pH should be between 7.0 and 7.5. I am curious to know if in performing an amniocentesis, testing of the amniotic fluid during pregnancy for older mothers, are they also checking the pH of the amniotic fluid? It is possible for the amniotic sac to have congestion or a slowing of its normal cleaning mechanism because of acidosis and excess proteins. Over time this can lead to the fluid being more toxic, affecting the baby that is immersed in and swallowing this fluid to help in organ development.

Shared Blood

Mother and baby share the same blood supply. The blood from the mother passes through the placenta to the baby. The placenta acts as a filter to further clean the blood for the baby. Can the mother be so acidic that the placenta gets overwhelmed and spills acidic waste and proteins into the blood supply of the baby? I believe the placenta, under normal healthy circumstances, will help keep blood pH and excess proteins under control for the baby. Many of the new mothers I collected saliva and urine test data from were severely acidic, below 5.5 with a few as low as 5.1. In these extreme cases of over acidity the placenta can become overwhelmed and congested leading to more acidic waste and proteins building in the organ and spilling into the baby's blood supply.

Studies show that 25% of pregnant woman experience some acid related problems daily, 50% experience some acid problems during their pregnancy. In my research I have realized most pregnant mothers are severely acidic which slows their lymphatic system allowing fluid, proteins and acid waste to build in the mother (preeclampsia) and in the fetus. Recently a mother of an autistic child informed me that her placenta had an extreme amount of calcification when her child was born. That calcification was due to a buildup of proteins, minerals and waste that could have overflowed into the fetus's blood supply and brain.

If proteins build in the eyes of the fetus it may have vision problems or be blind, if proteins build in the nerves or muscles of the fetus Muscular Dystrophy may develop, if waste builds in the lungs the child may have cystic fibrosis or asthma, if waste builds in the brain hydrocephalus, ADD, Batten disease, Asperger's, Autism or other diseases of the brain may develop. Not understanding how being too acidic negatively affects the lymphatic system, some mothers are unknowingly congesting their baby in the womb.

These newborns are being affected by a toxic tissue acidosis that traps excess proteins in the body and brain. To blame genetics for the newborns illnesses is easy. When we understand the emerging science of this undetected tissue acidosis and its negative affect on the lymphatic system an answer becomes evident.

Colic and Stiff Babies, Mom Beware

I have heard many explanations for colic; gas, an immature digestive system, or inhaling air from crying. It is basically over acidic intestinal tissue that may have started in the womb and made worse by sour breast milk or protein laden infant formula.

Over the years, I have seen many tight babies with colic who had trouble turning their heads to one side (tortocollis). At that time I didn't understand what caused it. Over acidity and excess proteins can make the infant toxic and tight. Acidic muscles that are very contracted in the body and neck are pulling the infant's head to one side. After a few sessions of CranioSacral and Lymph Drainage Therapy the infant becomes looser and calmer. At our wellness center we teach parents a few techniques to do at home in order to help relax the baby and improve lymphatic flow and cerebrospinal fluid circulation.

10 Tips for a Healthy Pregnancy

1. Mom and Dad start detoxing and nutritionally building your body in the months prior to conception.
2. Lay off or reduce processed foods, beef, coffee and sodas.
3. Eat a Greener diet - more fruits and vegetables, small portions of grains, chicken and fish.
4. Increase your circulation – Daily light exercise, deep breathing, good posture and drink more mineralized water.
5. Reduce Stress - Monthly massage or relaxing alternative therapy, meditation, laugh more.
6. Not even one puff of a cigarette or one drink of alcohol.
7. Be extremely careful during the first eight weeks while the fetus is being formed. No Meds if possible.
8. If you begin to swell and have high blood pressure, see your health care practitioner and start steps 2-5.
9. Know and understand your saliva and urine pH.
10. Manually activate your lymphatic system.

CHAPTER TEN

A New Look At Disease

What Needs To Be Reexamined

By missing the basis of most disease, which is a toxic tissue acidosis, a malfunctioning lymphatic system and protein proliferation, the medical community is working hard to try and help you but they are not seeing the real cause of disease. They are missing two major pieces of information that are important in keeping your cells healthy and free of disease. When you have any medical procedure or take a medication, the surgeon or pharmaceutical company is taking for granted that your tissue pH is in a healthy range. When your blood pH is tested it is almost always in the region of 7.37 - 7.43. Almost 43 - 51% of the individuals in my studies, where urine and saliva are used tested below 5.5. That means many people are almost 100 times more acidic than they are expected to be. Over acidity is a serious problem that is not properly tested for.

Many medications are intended to work in a set pH range. Can this undetected super acidity affect a person taking medications? Can it have life threatening consequences for a person about to have anesthesia and medications in the operating room? The effects of many of our medications and medical procedures on tissue pH and the lymphatic system are unknown and need to be evaluated by the government and medical community. This emerging science and missed information is critical to your understanding of health and disease prevention.

I am mentioning a few things here that need to be reexamined. Truly everything regarding health care, especially medications, needs to be reevaluated with this new understanding of acid-alkaline balance and the lymphatic system. My hope is that by writing this, researchers will then begin the process of including this emerging science in their paradigm of medicine. Once you include a toxic tissue acidosis and the lymphatic system to your existing medical paradigm, many of your unanswered questions and medical mysteries become apparent.

War on Cancer

President Nixon declared war on cancer in 1971 with the National Cancer Act. At that time, one in twenty individuals were diagnosed with cancer. In 2003 one in three individuals would be diagnosed with cancer in their lifetime. Next time you are with your family or friends look around the room, one out of three of you will be diagnosed with cancer in your lifetime. It's a scary scenario. Something is missing that is not allowing us to see how cancer and other diseases truly work. That missing key is tissue acidosis and its negative affect on your lymphatic system. While we are searching for a cure, we need to educate the public about internal balance and the lymphatic systems role in prevention of disease.

According to Felicia Drury Kliment, adjunct professor at City College in New York and author of The Acid-Alkaline Balance Diet, "Clearly the prevention of cancer should begin with removing from the body acidic wastes that turn normal cells into cancerous ones." When circulation is impeded over many months or even years, the stagnant fluid in the tissues becomes toxic and goes through chemical changes as toxicity builds. The cells in this area die or mutate to live off the toxic, anaerobic (lacking oxygen) environment. This is the basis of the disease process, whether it is a mole, Candida or cancer. Change the cellular environment in the affected area by activating the lymphatic system to move waste out and bring in oxygen and nutrition, and the disease process can change.

Get Out and Move

Lance Armstrong, seven-time winner of the Tour De France and a cancer survivor, had testicular cancer that spread to his abdomen, lungs and brain. Exercise is good for you, extreme amounts of exercise, as in Lance's case, can deplete the body of alkaline minerals creating an imbalance in the body. Besides cutting edge medical care, I believe a large part of his recovery was due in part to increased circulation. While healing, Lance got right back on his bike and trained, increasing his circulation of oxygen, nutrition and medications through his tissues. The increased circulation also cleaned his body of excess cellular debris from the cancer treatments.

Don't Wait, Take Action!

A few times I have heard from patients that when they were first told they had pre-cancerous cells or a small lump they were told to wait three months to see if further treatment was necessary. If I were in this situation I would get a second opinion, immediately. Then take action to change the cellular environment in the area with the pre-cancerous cells or lump. Balance your body with extra nutritional support, increase your lymph flow and blood circulation.

Cancer

It's very important to realize that cancers begin in the cells, which make up your entire body. Leukemia is a cancer that starts in tissues that are made of blood forming cells, such as bone marrow. In leukemia, damaged white blood cells are being over produced. Their large numbers crowd out the red blood cells, leading to anemia. The hallmark signs of leukemia are recurring infections, anemia, and easy bruising. Other signs include an enlarged spleen or liver, fatigue, pallor (paleness in the face), headaches, low grade fever, swollen lymph nodes, confusion, bleeding, mouth sores, or skin rashes.

Lymphoma is the most common blood cancer. It affects the lymphoid tissues of the body. The signs of lymphoma include swollen lymph nodes in the neck, underarm or groin, constant fatigue, unexplained weight-loss, night sweats, itchy rashes and reddened patches on the skin. In both of these diseases white blood cells become malignant and multiply, overcrowding the healthy cells. As these excess cells accumulate in your tissues, including your bones, lymphatic system and organs, congestion begins. This can interfere with circulation through your bones and the production of healthy blood cells and the removal of damaged or dead cells. The signs of both cancers are also signs and symptoms of a toxic tissue acidosis. Cancer begins in any part of the body where circulation is limited.

Patient Profile: Julia R.

Julia R. is a music teacher who is loved by her students; she is also a cancer survivor. She found our center searching for CranioSacral Therapy (CST) to treat herself to some relaxing and rejuvenating bodywork after making it through chemotherapy and a lumpectomy for breast cancer. She actually thought it would be a one-time occurrence. She felt so energetic and alive after that first session she came back once a week for a few months, then bimonthly for over five years. Julia started radiation treatments at the same time she started CST and credits the therapy for keeping her feeling well during her weeks of radiation treatments. When Julia's upper arm began to swell due to lymph nodes being removed in her underarm, she had to have Lymphedema Therapy and started to wear a compression sleeve to control the excess fluid. Months after her Lymphedema Therapy, I used Lymph Drainage Therapy to reroute the pooling lymph to more efficient areas of main lymph nodes. With regular lymph drainage therapy, self-drainage and the information in this book, especially a more alkaline diet and systemic enzymes, Julia was able to stop wearing her compression garment.

Julia is one of my patients that has really learned the importance of acid-alkaline balance, nutritional supplementation, exercise and maintenance with lymphatic activation to help keep her arm from swelling, and to prevent future disease. She comes in every two weeks for a one-hour session. We decide what she needs by how she is feeling. If she is stressed we do more work on her craniosacral system and less work on the lymphatic system. Since she has had lymph nodes removed we always open her main areas of lymph nodes and reroute her lymph in that area to more efficient lymph nodes. When Julia feels congested we do a few Lymphatic Cellular Detox Massage sessions.

Stress can create a great deal of acid in your body, which will impede your lymphatic system and you become congested. Julia has become very aware of her lymph flow. Recently at the beginning of one of our sessions she told me she felt like one big mass of lymph, very congested. It had only been a few days since I had seen Julia, so I wondered how she could have become so congested. She said everything had been the same, her 80/20 diet, water consumption, exercise, systemic enzymes and alkalizing supplements. As the session began Julia realized she had just bought a new car the day before. The transaction was very stressful for her. Stress can slow or stop your lymph flow within seconds. A few months before, Julia also told me she felt very lymph congested and tight. After she mentally checked her routine for the past few days at that time to see what may have been different, she realized she had run out of her systemic enzymes about four days prior. Proteolytic systemic enzymes help keep your lymph flow moving by lysing (eating) excess proteins that are clogging the body. Without them you congest easily.

Julia's story holds a warning to anyone who has had breast cancer and nodes removed and those with Lymphedema. For five years Julia did not have to wear a compression garment to control her swollen arm due to the many proactive steps like lymph drainage therapy, a more alkaline diet, systemic enzymes and self-lymphatic activation. When she went for a colonoscopy, a blood pressure cuff was left on her affected arm for the procedure. Since that time she has found it difficult to control her Lymphedema and is now wearing her compression garment again. Lymphedema can start the day after surgery to 30 or more years down the road as waste and proteins continue to fill and congest the existing nodes in the area. If you have had nodes removed or Lymphedema never have your blood pressure taken or injections in the affected arm and always wear a compression garment when flying.

Acid is Aging

We all age differently. Your skin shows how well you age. Some of us age very gracefully and some of us age very aggressively, with thin, wrinkled skin. Why this happens is dependent on how healthy or how toxic your skin is. What can be more aging to your skin than acid flowing through it? My wife had our first child one month before her 40th birthday and our second child at 41. She doesn't have a stretch mark on her body. She took 30 nutritional supplements a day. Many of those were herbs rich in minerals, like alfalfa. If your skin is acidic it interferes with collagen's ability to allow your skin to stretch and then return without leaving stretch marks. Acidosis makes your skin less elastic and thin. There are many young mothers who have stretch marks on their abdomen. This occurred because their tissues were overly acidic.

To age gracefully you need daily exercise, deep breathing, water and alkalizing supplements to balance the acid in your body. Lymphatic activation can specifically increase lymph flow and blood circulation in your skin. Be sure to take alkalizing supplements. Minerals must be available to flow around and into your cells for skin to become healthier and alive again. When your lymphatic system is damaged or acidic, toxins and dead cells can build in your skin. To have healthy skin you need good circulation and healthy cells.

Alzheimer's Disease

Alzheimer's is stealing the minds of seniors. According to the Merck Manual, 4.5 Million Americans have Alzheimer's. Recent research shows that B-amyloid (a misfolded protein) and neurofibrillary tangles of tau protein, both are parts of cells, are building up in the brain of Alzheimer's patients. The key word is protein. Researchers say these proteins look similar to staples. When there is a single layer of these staples, as in the normal aging process, there are no problems with the ability to think. As these proteins begin to double, triple and quadruple, we begin having problems thinking. Newer studies are finding that brains of Alzheimer's patients have increased levels of fibrin.

The lymphatic system helps to recapture large proteins like fibrin that have escaped from the blood supply. When it is malfunctioning due to an acidic pH, proteins can build in the tissues of the brain clogging microvascular circulation and nerve synapses, leading to a loss of cognitive function. To help prevent Alzheimer's you need to rebalance your body. Activating the lymphatic system will help to remove acidic waste and proteins out of your cerebrospinal fluid and brain. In Lymphatic Cellular Detox Massage we concentrate on whole body circulation by activating the lymphatic system to increase circulation in the body and brain. It is very effective at enhancing overall circulation, to nourish the cells and to help remove excess proteins and waste. Another way to increase circulation is by taking systemic enzymes. These enzymes are super foods and are an important part to keeping proteins from building in the body and brain. Systemic enzymes have the ability to cross the blood/brain barrier to help lyse (breakdown) excess proteins in the brain.

Obesity

According to recent statistics, 2/3 of our population is overweight. That's 135 million people. The current explanation why we gain weight is simple; we are using less energy than we consume. They also write obesity is elusive, involving the regulation of body weight, primarily fat, in the body. How this regulation is achieved is not fully understood. An undetected acidosis is why many in our nation are overweight. After getting married I slowly gained about 40 pounds. For almost twenty years I yo-yo dieted. I would lose weight on a diet and gain it back when I stopped the diet. Once I learned about acidosis I lost the weight in a few months and have not gained it back. When you are more alkaline your lymphatic system can pick up fibrin, acid waste, cellular debris, lipids and minerals which combine together to form fat in your tissues or organs.

New Research Links Damaged Lymph Vessels to Obesity

Two new studies have linked damaged lymph vessels to the accumulation of fat and adult-onset obesity. These studies are ground breaking and show that the lymphatics play a major role in obesity.

Research 1: A group of researchers from St. Jude Children's Research Hospital in Memphis, Tennessee inactivated a gene called Prox1. This gene is required for the healthy formation of lymph vessels. This inactivation led to abnormal lymph leakage from mispatterned and ruptured lymph vessels. The researchers identified lymphatic vasculature dysfunction as a cause of adult-onset obesity. Natasha L. Harvey, R. Sathish Srinivasan, Miriam E. Dillard, Nicole C. Johnson, Marlys H. Witte, Kelli Boyd, Mark W. Sleeman & Guillermo Oliver, Lymphatic vascular defects promoted by Prox1 haploinsufficiency cause adult-onset obesity, Nature Genetics 37, 1072 –1081 (2005)

Research 2: At the Center for Transgene Technology and Gene Therapy in Leuven, Belgium researchers inactivated the same Prox1 gene, as above, revealing a link between fat deposition and lymph fluid. These researchers agree these findings bring the lymphatic system into the focus of obesity research. Martin Schneider, Edward M. Conway & Peter Carmeliet, Lymph Makes You Fat, Nature Genetics 37, 1023 – 1024 (2005)

The lymphatic system picks up milky white lymph from the intestines called chyle. Normally the lymph is a clear, sometimes yellowish liquid. It turns white when it absorbs lipids and fats from your intestines. If you are acidic your lymphatic system is not picking up lipids such as cholesterol and fats like triglycerides efficiently, trapping them in your tissues with fibrin, cellular debris and minerals. This is what accumulates to form what we call fat. This waxy fat and cellular debris can become like glue in your tissues further limiting microcirculation around your cells. Cellulite is an extreme case of this protein and debris congested tissue.

After trying every diet for almost twenty years, I was amazed that when I started alkalizing my system (eating 90% alkaline and 10% acid) and started taking alkalizing supplements, systemic enzymes as well as exercising, I lost weight quickly. I can bloat and gain weight in a few days if I eat more acid foods. Proper balance is the key. If I have a party to go to on a weekend or I am vacationing, I enjoy what I want to eat but balance it with more fruits, vegetables, nutritional support and exercise in an effort to keep my body more alkaline and free of excess proteins and acid. It's about creating balance.

Arteriosclerosis, Angina and Heart Attacks

Heart disease and clogging of the arteries may be due, in many cases, to acid damaging the heart cells and eating away at the blood vessel walls. The body's defense is to send fibrin, a protein that looks like pieces of yarn, to repair the damaged vessels. The excess protein builds up with parts of dead cells and mixes with collagen, cholesterol, phospholipids, heavy metals and other cellular debris to make plaque, which builds on the artery walls. The body is trying to repair damage to the vessel wall by creating a patch, as waste and proteins build in your arteries, it may lead to a decrease in circulation, or a clog that may lead to heart disease or a heart attack. The term arteriosclerosis means scarring of the artery. This scarring occurs due to proteins like fibrin and parts of dead cells building up in the tissues or vessels.

Research shows that 50% of heart attack victims have normal cholesterol levels. New research is looking at inflammation as a cause in arteriosclerosis. A heart attack may be due to inflammation from acidity and a malfunctioning lymphatic system in the vessel wall or heart tissue creating a spasm or clot that stops blood flow. The vasa vasorum, a tiny set of vessels including lymphatic vessels in the blood vessel wall may play an important role in inflammation and possible spasms of the blood vessel or heart tissue. If your lymphatic system is congested, circulation is slowed and may create a toxic backup in the tiny lymph vessels in the blood vessel wall or heart. This allows the tissues to become overly acidic and protein filled, where it may spasm or clog the vessel or heart, limiting circulation and damaging the cells that make up the vessel wall or heart. Continued lack of circulation can lead to inflammation, possible further fibrosis and death of cells in the involved area.

According to the medical literature angina pain occurs when oxygen demand exceeds the ability of the coronary arteries to supply oxygenated blood. Upon an autopsy, patients with long-standing angina have extensive coronary atherosclerosis and patchy myocardial fibrosis. If the lymph flow is impeded in the heart tissue, oxygen cannot get to the heart cells efficiently and proteins cannot be removed efficiently, creating angina and fibrosis. The heart becomes more constricted, limiting its ability to pump blood and oxygen.

Arterial Hypertension: High Blood Pressure

This is another ailment affecting us in great numbers. About one in three Americans suffer with high blood pressure and the increased risk of kidney disease, cardiovascular disease and suffering a stroke or heart attack. Blood pressure (BP) is considered high if it is 140/90 mmHg (millimeter of mercury) and above. The 140 mmHg is the maximum force exerted on the arterial wall at peak cardiac output. The 90 mmHg is the resting heart rate and the minimum force put on an arterial wall. The primary reason for high blood pressure is unknown. A combination of problems may be working together to cause high blood pressure. When you are diagnosed with hypertension, your high blood pressure can be caused by vasoconstriction (blood vessels that have tightened), obstructions such as a buildup of arteriosclerotic plaque on a vessel wall, kidney problems or increased levels of sodium in the cell. One of the hall-marks of hypertension is nephrosclerosis, which is another term for scarring and hardening of the kidney. When you are overly acidic your urine will test at 5.0, this means overly acidic fluid is passing through the kidneys, this acidity can cause the organ to constrict allowing excess proteins to become trapped in the kidney, making them hard and scarred, limiting blood flow further.

The kidney is made up of structural units called nephrons. It is a tiny tubule consisting of a group of capillaries called the glomerulus. The nephron filters the blood by several processes, concentrating the waste and minerals as water and other dissolved substances pass. As these tiny capillaries become filled with debris, the kidney becomes less efficient. Just like dirty air conditioner filters limit air flow. The kidneys play an important role in alkalizing the body, eliminating wastes, regulating blood volume and blood pressure. It takes pressure to move blood through the kidney to make urine. Large molecules such as proteins and blood cells that are too big to pass through the glomerulus of the nephron begin to congest the kidney. To keep blood flowing through the protein congested kidneys, the heart must pump harder (high blood pressure) to push fluid through the kidneys .

Over acidity creates protein proliferation. Sclerosis or scarring can be caused by the buildup of fibrin, parts of dead cells and other proteins that form scar tissue and cause limited circulation in a tissue or organ. In hypertension you may also have sclerosis of the arteries of the brain, heart or legs. If you follow some of the ideas in this book you will feel a difference in a matter of weeks, it may take a few months to a year to increase your circulation to help clean proteins and acid waste from your tissues and organs. High blood pressure medications work by either, removing water and sodium or limit the ability of the heart to pump. These medications do nothing to remove acid waste and proteins that are causing the problem.

Diabetes

Sixteen million Americans may be suffering with diabetes. There are two studies on the Internet, one from 1981 and one from 1985, that show insulin action in the cell is severely impaired by an acidic pH.

pH/Insulin Research

"The influence of pH and 3-hydroxybutyrate on insulin binding and action has been studied in cultured human fibroblast. When the pH of the incubation medium was decreased from 7.6 to 6.8, insulin stimulation of glycogen synthase and total glucose uptake was decreased. The decreased pH induced both an increase in the insulin concentration for half-maximal response, and a decrease in maximal responsiveness...The data show that insulin action is impaired at lower pH. The decreased sensitivity is probably related to the decrease in insulin binding affinity at lower pH..."

H Hidaka, BV Howard, F Ishibashi, FC Kosmakos, JW Craig, PH Bennett and J Larner, Effect of pH and 3-hydroxybutyrate on insulin binding and action in cultured human fibroblasts, Diabetes, 1981, Vol 30, Issue 5 402-406

"we examined the effectiveness of insulin during and after 48 h of exposure of cultured 3T3-L1 adipocytes to low pH and ketoacids. In the "acute" stage, lowering of physiologic pH (pH 7.4) to pH 6.9 induced a decrease in insulin binding (50%), which was due to a decrease in the rate of association. Concomitantly, the insulin sensitivity was decreased (ninefold)... These postbinding alterations induced by low pH could be reversed by culturing the cells at physiologic pH for another 48 h.

JP Van Putten, T Wieringa and HM Krans, Low pH and ketoacids induce insulin receptor binding and postbinding alterations in cultured 3T3 adipocytes, Diabetes, Vol 34, Issue 8 744-750

In the study from 1981 researchers used a fibroblast, which is a cell that forms the basis of connective tissue. Fibroblasts can become bone cells, fat cells or smooth muscle cells. In the study from 1985 researchers used an adipocyte (fat cell). Researchers placed these cells in a slightly alkaline solution with a pH of 7.4 - 7.6. When they lowered the pH of the solution to 6.8 - 6.9, which is only slightly acidic, insulin action of the cell was dramatically impaired. One study showed a 50% reduction in insulin binding. Only 7% of those in my study were in a healthy pH range above 6.5.

In these studies the insulin action of the cell is impaired with only a few tenths of a change into the acid side of the pH scale. Over 43-51% of the individuals in my study were below 5.5. This is 100 times more acidic than the culture used in the studies and can dramatically negatively affect insulin action.

Important Point

The study from 1985 went a step further. After returning the pH of the cellular environment to a healthy alkaline environment of 7.4 - 7.6, the changes in insulin action that were induced by the acidic pH, were reversed. Within 48 hours the cell was back to normal insulin activity.

The above statement shows that diabetics need to return to a more alkaline pH to increase insulin action and move towards becoming healthy. Diabetes is about insulin action of the cell! Dehydration and an acidic pH can cause excess proteins to build around and in your cells and tissues, like the pancreas, which can damage cells and limit their ability to function. The pancreas, when hydrated and functioning optimally, plays an important role in buffering excess acid from your system. The lymphatic system is responsible for removing proteins and maintaining the health of your cells and organs. Your ability to utilize insulin depends on circulation around and in your cells, especially the islet cells of the pancreas. Can type 1 diabetes begin in the womb with cellular waste filling the pancreas? Acidity and excess proteins can damage the pancreas and other cells that deal with insulin in the womb.

Headaches and Migraines

If you suffer from migraines it often starts with your shoulder and neck muscles becoming tight. This occurs as congested fluid around your muscles in your neck and shoulders becomes more acidic. We learned about the Lymph/Brain Connection where almost 48% of your cerebrospinal fluid is absorbed by the lymphatic system. As your lymphatic system becomes more congested and toxic, it slows. This creates a backup of cerebrospinal fluid, raising intracranial pressure which may be the pain, pressure or throbbing that you feel with a headache. I believe that as this pressure builds it can put pressure in or on the optic nerve, which may be migraines with auras or visual disturbances.

Autoimmune Disorders

Autoimmune disorders are conditions thought to be caused by an immune response against the body's own tissues. The result can be the destruction of body tissues, enlargement of an organ or changes in organ function. There are over 80 autoimmune disorders like arthritis, Multiple Sclerosis and lupus. Symptoms include joint pain, fatigue, dizziness, bleeding and skin sores. This missed overly acidic internal environment plays a major role in autoimmune diseases. Acid is corroding or destroying cells and tissues in the body.

Multiple Sclerosis (MS)

Multiple sclerosis is an autoimmune disease, the exact cause is unknown. Most researchers believe that the damage to myelin, which surrounds and protects the nerves like insulation, is from an abnormal immune response where the body is attacking its own tissue. This creates bare spots and scarred areas along the nerve which interfere with nerve conduction. An acidic environment and excess proteins may be damaging the myelin around the nerves. Acidity in the tiny lymph vessel (vaso vasorum) in the nerve may play a role in creating inflammation that could damage the myelin of the nerve.

In a 2004 study from University of California San Diego, Katerina Akassoglous, Ph.D the study's first author writes, "Multiple sclerosis is a nervous system disease with vascular damage, resulting from leakage of blood proteins, including fibrin, into the brain... Our study shows that fibrin facilitates the initiation of the inflammatory response in the nervous system and contributes to nerve tissue damage in an animal model of the disease."

MS patients experience muscle weakness beginning in their arms or legs. They also have difficulty with coordination, balance, bladder and bowel dysfunction and diminished vision. In the worst cases, MS can produce partial or complete paralysis. Most with MS also have numbness or the sensation of "pins and needles." This is also a sign of Amyloidosis where proteins can become trapped in any part of the body including the nerves. Many with MS experience pain, speech impediments, tremors, and dizziness. Some experience cognitive impairments such as difficulties with concentration, attention, and memory. Another common symptom is depression. These are all symptoms of acidosis.

Muscular Dystrophy (MD)

Muscular Dystrophy is a group of genetic, hereditary muscle diseases that cause progressive muscle weakness. Many individuals with the same genetic makeup get MD's of different severity. Symptoms include progressive muscle wasting, weakness, loss of muscle function, enlarged calf muscles, calf pain, joint tightness, obesity, cataracts, frontal baldness and mental impairment. All these symptoms are acid related. If the lymph cannot flow through the muscles or nerves to complete circulation, the muscles and nerves become acidic, protein filled and weak which can result in pain or loss of function. The enlarged calf muscle is congested and filled with stagnant, acidic fluid due to congested lymph nodes above the calf . Most types of MD are not muscle specific they are multi-system disorders with manifestations throughout the body including the heart, gastrointestinal and nervous systems, endocrine glands, skin, eyes and other organs. The acid waste and proteins that are building in the muscles and nerves are also building in other parts of the body.

ALS / Lou Gehrig's Disease

In the 1930's Lou Gehrig a New York Yankees baseball great was stricken with ALS. His name has become synonymous with the disease. Amyotrophic lateral sclerosis (ALS) is a motor neuron disease that is progressive and often rapid disease that attacks the nerve cells (neurons) responsible for controlling voluntary muscle activity. Symptoms begin with muscle weakness and atrophy, fasciculations, muscle cramping then respiratory muscle weakness. Since the muscles aren't receiving nerve stimulation they weaken and waste away.

As the disease progresses, breathing without a respirator becomes difficult. Eventually patients will be unable to walk or stand, or use their hands and arms. Often the disease does not affect the mind of the person with ALS, although some may experience problems with thinking, depression, and dementia. Most patients with ALS die of respiratory failure or pneumonia. If you begin to have muscle weakness or fasciculations don't wait for a diagnosis which may take up to a year. Immediately change your lifestyle and follow the steps to balance your body and activate your lymphatics. Since this a nervous system disorder, see a chiropractor to address the spinal cord and nerves.

Patient Profile: Brian H.

I didn't know much about ALS until I met Brian H, a veteran Phoenix police officer with Bulbar ALS. I was very fortunate to meet Brian, he taught me a great deal about ALS. When I first met Brian he was in great shape physically except his speech and ability to swallow were beginning to become affected due to the disease. His left hand was beginning to weaken and atrophy. Bulbar ALS begins in the cranial nerves that innervate the mouth and throat. As the disease progresses to the limbs, swallowing becomes difficult and the vagus nerve that innervates the heart, lungs and stomach becomes affected.

Brian's biggest complaint at our first meeting was severe tightness in his TMJ muscles and a popping sound when he opened his jaw. Brian was a great patient to work with because he was pro-active in learning all he could about ALS and was already taking many supplements. Within a few weeks of combined sessions of CranioSacral Therapy and Lymph Drainage Therapy Brian's jaw was no longer tight or popping. During over two years of sessions I saw that Lymph Drainage Therapy and CranioSacral Therapy were able to help in reducing and eliminating contractures, help with depression, slow the progression of the disease but did nothing to stop the disease.

ALS is thought to be brought on by several factors, including a virus; exposure to neurotoxins or heavy metals; DNA defects; immune system abnormalities; and enzyme abnormalities. After meeting Brian and hearing his story I believe an accumulation of trauma and protein in his cranial nerves, over years or decades began his disease. While speaking with Brian's mom, she told me about a fall Brian had taken as a young boy. He was running and fell on his chin so hard that his head snapped back and he almost bit through his tongue. This fall as a young boy, snapping the head back, may have been the first damage that crimped or damaged Brian's spinal cord or cranial nerves. This damage could have limited circulation and allowed cellular waste and fibrin to build in the region of the cranial nerves for years leading to ALS.

As a young adult Brian had many viruses which can lead to excess proteins in the body. Later as a police officer Brian responded to emergencies many times during a shift, creating higher levels of stress hormones that could have played a role. Brian chewed tobacco for over a decade which could lead to more tissue damage and excess fibrin in the area from the constant irritation of the chewing tobacco. He was also a sharp shooter and remembers having his neck in an awkward position for hours while looking down his rifle scope. Even the toxic fumes from shooting at the rifle range for hours could have an affect. All of these add up to an accumulation of circumstances that could lead to a buildup of protein that damaged and scarred Brian's cranial nerves. According to medical texts in amyotrophic lateral sclerosis the nerves become "scarred and hardened." That scarring is caused by a buildup of proteins, fibrin, toxins and other debris. Most nerve problems are caused by fibrosis or scarring.

Fibromyalgia

Fibromyalgia is a chronic disease that affects mostly women. Between three to six million people in the United States are affected. Symptoms include numerous tender and painful spots on the body, debilitating fatigue, headaches and migraines, irritable bowel, restless leg syndrome, dry eyes and mouth, concentration problems, skin sensitivities, rashes, arthritis, anxiety, depression, dizziness, vision problems, the inability to think clearly, and impaired memory. Fibromyalgia is a circulation problem similar to arthritis, where acid waste and proteins become trapped in the tissues, skin, muscles, ligaments and tendons of the body. I have seen many patients with fibromyalgia improve by following the steps in this book to balance the body and activate the lymphatic system.

Osteoporosis

Osteoporosis is a bone wasting disease that affects 10 million people in the United States. According to the American Journal of Clinical Nutrition, the University of California, San Francisco, conducted a seven-year study of 9,000 women to study the effects of low pH or chronic acidosis on bone loss. The researchers found that women who have chronic acidosis are at a greater risk for bone loss than those who have normal pH levels. They believe that today's high acid diet is connected to the prevalence of hip fractures among middle-aged women. Osteoporosis was once thought to be a disease of old age. Now teenagers are beginning to be diagnosed with osteopenia, the beginning stage of osteoporosis, teens are very acidic. The blood will steal calcium from your bones, weakening them, to buffer the excess acid in the blood. Diets including more vegetables are alkalizing and can enhance calcium retention in the body. Exercise, especially strength training, has been shown to build bone mass.

Polycystic Diseases

Polycystic means to have more than one cyst. This can occur with breast cysts, cirrhosis of the liver, polycystic kidney disease (PKD) and ovarian cysts. I will discuss the possible cause of PKD but it also relates to the liver, ovaries and other areas where cysts can form. Let's take a look at Polycystic Kidney Disease (PKD) and see how a simple imbalance can negatively affect organs. Over acidity in an organ can impede the ability of the lymphatic system to remove fluid and proteins, creating pockets of stagnant fluid and proteins. In PKD, fluid-filled cysts form in the kidneys. These cysts can be numerous and grow very large, crowding out the kidney and making it unable to function normally. Cysts can often form in multiple organs at the same time. This shows us that cirrhosis or PKD is not organ specific. When you look at a picture of PKD, the kidney has many clear fluid filled cysts on its surface and in the organ itself. Being familiar with the lymphatic system's role in allowing circulation to move through the tissues and more specifically, through the interstitial spaces (spaces around your cells), I immediately understood that these fluid filled cysts could only be trapped interstitial fluid. The lymphatic system is an overflow mechanism for the circulatory system, when the lymphatic system is congested fluid builds in the tissue or organ. Remember, the lymphatic system is responsible for picking up the 2-10% of the fluid that is left behind in the tissues or organs. If the lymphatic system is unable to pick up the leftover fluid, it can build in the organ and become toxic, fluid filled cysts. Lymph Drainage Therapy can be very specific in increasing circulation in or around organs to relieve this buildup of fluid. Increasing your circulation using lymphatic activation, alkalizing products, and systemic enzymes are very important for helping to open lymph flow in the organs.

Aneurysm and Neuroma's

Aneurisms are a very common problem affecting many people. It is a bulging out of a blood vessel wall. It forms where the wall has weakened and can become a life-threatening situation if the ballooning vessel bursts. It occurs primarily in the brain and abdomen. A neuroma is a bulging out of a nerve wall. I believe the vasa vasourum (or tiny vessels in the vessel) especially the lymph vessel in the blood vessel or nerve can become toxic and congested. This can cause inflammation and weaken the outer layer of the blood vessel or nerve wall. As excess fluid, acidic waste and proteins that are not picked up by the lymphatic system build in the vessel or nerve wall, the weakened area can balloon out or burst.

Anorexia Nervosa

Anorexia nervosa usually occurs in adolescence or young adulthood. It is more common in females. It is an eating disorder where an individuals image of themselves is distorted. They may see themselves as overweight when in actuality they are dangerously thin. They try to lose more weight by eating very little or over exercising. When you starve the body or over exercise you create excess acid in the body that can create excess proteins that can congest the organs. Anorexia is most common among teen girls, but about 10 percent of teens with anorexia are boys. Studies have shown that teen athlets are at a higher risk for eating disorders, about one-third of teen girls who are athletes show some tendencies toward anorexia.

As an individual becomes acidic, their lymphatic system constricts and their organs, including the endocrine system and brain, become filled with cellular acid waste and proteins limiting their function. This could lead to the many symptoms associated with anorexia like fatigue, lowered white blood cell count, reduced immune function, hair loss, feeling of pins and needles, depression, pallid complexion, creaky joints, edema in ankles, feeling cold, dry skin, headaches, osteoporosis and bruising.

The abdominal discomfort or pain often felt by those with eating disorders may have to do with a congested cisterna chyli, 3 lymphatic vessels that are located by the right rib cage. When these vessels become congested acidic fluid fills the digestive system creating fullness and pain. When I look at all the above symptoms of eating disorders I immediately connect them to an overly acidic body and malfunctioning lymphatic system.

Helping Addictions

In diseases like alcohol or drug addiction understanding how to balance your body is of the utmost importance in recovery. When you have over used alcohol i.e., beer, wine or hard liquor and have used drugs to excess the internal body becomes severely acidic. The alcohol or drugs actually slow your body's ability to clean itself by creating acidity. This impedes your lymphatic system and negatively affect every system in the body including the brain and how you feel mentally. The beverage of choice for most recovering addicts is coffee which is very acid forming in the body and can affect the way you feel and think. A better choice is water.

We can help recovering addicts by educating them on balance, how lifestyle choices like diet, exercise, drinking mineralized water, stress reduction and self-lymphatic activation can imrove how they feel and think. To help in recovery seek help from Alcoholics Annonymous (AA) or Narcotics Annonymous (NA) and begin following the 5 Steps to Balance your Body and Activate your Lymphatic System in the following chapters. Be aware that as you begin eating more alkaline foods, drinking more water and deep breathing you may experience a Healing Crisis for a few days. This is a sign your body is detoxing waste that has been trapped in your tissues and organs.

To help the haling crisis try three big handfuls of Epsom salt in a luke warm bath. A hot bath is too detoxing and may stress you more. Make sure you are well hydrated at all times, you should aalways have a water bottle with you at all times.

C-Reactive Protein / Fibrinogen – Excess Proteins

Excess proteins role in inflammation is being viewed as a contributing factor in many diseases like heart disease, stroke, high blood pressure, diabetes, lung disease and cancer. Testing for C-Reactive Protein (CRP) and fibrinogen are good indicators of inflammation in the body. CRP is produced by the liver and found in the blood. A C-Reactive Protein test can be used for measuring the levels of CRP in the blood. Higher levels of CRP can indicate inflammation of the walls of arteries. CRP is not normally found in blood tests of healthy individuals but increases during phases of acute systemic inflammation, after injuries or infection. As an infection or inflammation goes away and an injury heals the CRP in the blood disappears. Those who smoke, have high blood pressure, are overweight and do not exercise have higher CRP levels.

Fibrinogen is a protein that is also synthesized in the liver that plays a key role in blood clotting. Fibrinogen is a sticky, fibrous coagulant in the blood that appears to significantly increase the risk of heart attack and stroke. Fibrinogen is a precursor to fibrin which is meant to heal your injuries. Most acute heart attacks are now known to be due to acute thrombosis, or the sudden formation of a blood clot at the site of an atherosclerotic plaque. Fibrinogen promotes blood clotting; it makes sense that elevated fibrinogen levels would be associated with an increased risk of heart attack.

An increased level of CRP or fibrinogen in the blood may be indicative of undiagnosed inflammation. According to current research those with higher levels of CRP or fibrinogen can often reduce their levels by initiating lifestyle changes like those mentioned in this book, quit smoking, take a multivitamin, eat more nutritiously, and include healthy oils like olive oil and omega-3 fatty acids. Balancing the body and activating the lymphatics are the missing keys to removing excess proteins and inflammation in the body.

CHAPTER ELEVEN

A Further Look at Disease and Medicine

Inflammation – Lack of Circulation

I recently treated a young woman a few times for chronic neck and back pain that she had for almost a year. During that time she had a lot of emotional trauma, stress and a few automobile accidents. Her neck and shoulder muscles were extremely tight, like rocks. After a few sessions of increasing circulation in her lymphatic system and craniosacral system, the pain was gone. With improved lymph flow and blood circulation her neck and shoulder muscles relaxed again. After not seeing this woman for a year, she came in again with intense and debilitating neck pain. During our session she told me that months ago she had more intense stress and another automobile accident. Remember stress is very acid forming and constricting. I could feel that her neck and shoulder muscles had become hard again, fibrotic. She also told me she had been having a recurring infection in her mastoid bone (part of your skull by the base of the ear). Doctors were unable to control the infection with repeated rounds of antibiotics. She said that during the last procedure to control the infection they cut through her skin and drilled a hole in the mastoid bone in the back of her head. They said they were doing this to allow the infection to drain.

It had been three months since the surgery and when I felt the muscles and tissues by her mastoid, they were still very hot from the ongoing inflammation. This woman endured horrible pain and recurring infections for months. After our first session of increasing the circulation in her neck and shoulders, she told me before leaving that her neck was feeling much better already. By the second session her neck and shoulders were looser and her pain was much less. When I felt the tissues of the mastoid area the heat from the inflammation was barely perceivable. Infections occur due to lack of circulation. Antibiotics and surgery (drilling a hole in the head) create excess proteins and acidic waste that limit circulation further. You just can't drill a hole and hope for the best, lymphatic activation is needed to increase circulation in the area. When your tissues and organs become inflamed and fill with fibrin and other proteins they become fibrotic (hard) and circulation is impeded. You need to activate the lymphatics in the affected area to remove proteins and reduce inflammation.

Organ Transplant

Having an organ transplant is difficult for the recipient but it also puts hardships on the families involved. Often a family member will donate part of a liver or full kidney. Most of the patients who are told they will need a new organ will have to wait a year or more for the donor organ and surgery. In that year or more they need to increase their circulation and change the pH of the affected area in order to ensure a better outcome with surgery. Most patients continue on and don't do anything but take medications like a blood thinner and wait for the surgery. Take action! What do you have to lose? Find a second doctor who understands acid-alkaline balance, lymphatic activation, systemic enzymes and the information in this book about increasing circulation. Please, don't just sit and wait. Your life and possibly the life of a loved one (who may be your donor) depend on your actions.

The importance of increasing circulation cannot be overstated. By learning to balance your body and to activate your lymphatics in the year or two you are waiting for an organ you can possibly eliminate enough protein and waste from your system so surgery may not be necessary. If the organ still needs to be replaced, at least the tissues surrounding the organ will be cleaner, more alkaline and have more blood and lymph flow to accept the new organ. In transplanting organs the lymphatic system is ignored; only the arteries and veins are reconnected. By not having a well-established lymphatic system, the new organ can fill with its own waste, especially fibrin and dead cells.

The missed lymphatic system may play a major role in organ rejection. After your surgery if you are not vigilant about acid-alkaline balance, water intake, increasing circulation daily, stress reduction and lymphatic activation your organ may fill with proteins and begin having problems.

Patient Profile: Josie M.

Inflammation can start from within us without outside influences such as trauma. Let me tell you about a very active 80-year old woman named Josie M. She had gone on a cruise with her husband and when they went to board the ship there was a long line. They didn't think to go to the front of the line or to ask for assistance. Two and a half hours later, and hardly able to stand, they boarded the ship and went to their room. That night Josie's calf was swollen. The next day it was hurting and more swollen. By the third day it was hot to the touch and had a small sore. The ship's doctor said she must have scraped herself and it had become infected.

Three months and multiple rounds of antibiotics later, the wound on her leg was not healing. A clear fluid seeped from the wound continually. This clear fluid (interstitial fluid) is meant to bathe and nourish your cells. When lymph flow becomes slowed or stopped due to an injury, surgery or infection, interstitial fluid pools at the wound site. This stagnant fluid can impede the ability of the wound to heal. Josie is a family relative and was eager to see if lymphatic activation could heal her three-month old wound. When Josie told me about her ordeal she said she didn't remember scraping her leg and that the sore had appeared after the swelling. If you have an undetected minor circulation problem, standing for long periods allows excess fluid to build in the legs. This stagnant fluid can become very toxic and protein filled beginning the inflammation process without outside influences. Within one week of two lymphatic activation sessions to increase her circulation, the wound had stopped seeping and was starting to scab over. It was completely healed within a month. For healing to occur in a tissue or organ we need to have complete circulation of lymph and blood.

Wounds That Won't Heal

There are entire departments within hospitals that deal exclusively with wound care, especially wounds that are slow to heal or are not healing at all. Lymphatic activation is very effective at enhancing circulation and healing wounds in only a few sessions.

Pre and Post Surgery

When an area has been damaged from trauma or surgery, the lymph and blood vessels become damaged. It has been shown in studies that it takes between seven to ten days for the lymphatic vessels to become re-established and functional after surgery or trauma. Regeneration of lymphatic vessels is complete after fourteen days. Blood vessels take twelve days to completely regenerate.

Lymph Drainage Therapy (LDT) before surgery, prepares the tissues by enhancing lymph flow to bring fresh blood to the tissues and to remove waste like fibrin and cellular waste. LDT after surgery helps to minimize inflammation, infection and speed recovery. It is best to have a series of lymphatic activation sessions completed a week prior to the surgery. This gives you time to build your system up before the surgery. Two days before surgery, have a gentle lymph drainage therapy session to open your lymph flow in the affected area. This will allow for good circulation after the procedure in order to lower your risk of inflammation and infection. As long as there are no complications, have another light LDT session 24-48 hours after surgery. Lymph drainage therapy is very effective in reducing edema (swelling), pain and inflammation from surgery or trauma. With lymph drainage therapy we can increase circulation in the wound by working far from the site of surgery. When excess protein builds in a scar it is called a keloid scar. These scars are heavier and thicker than a normal scar. LDT can reduce fibrin and protein buildup in the newly forming scar, this is especially important after facial or cosmetic surgery.

Burns

The few times I have worked on burn victims I was able to map the lymph flow around their wounds. The lymph flowed normally where there were no blisters. Wherever a blister formed, the lymph was flowing backwards into the blister. One burn victim had burned her hand with hot lasagna. A few days after her doctor visit there were a few blisters and the wound was very red and wet. We drained her underarm, arm and areas around the wound. The patient said the burn felt better, less pressure, immediately after we started to drain her arm. At the site of the blisters I corrected the lymph flow and the next day the blisters were gone. The wound even looked drier and healthier and within a week the scabs were beginning to reduce. The wound healed exceptionally fast.

When the skin is severely damaged by a burn, the lymph vessels may be damaged or burned away. A lymph drainage therapist can help create new tissue channels to route fluid from under the new skin or skin graft to help fluid circulation through the new tissue. This increased circulation may increase the ability of the graft to take.

Brain and Spinal Cord Injuries

Brain and spinal cord injuries affect millions of Americans annually. Swelling in the brain or spinal cord is a major concern after brain injury or surgery. If swelling in the brain cannot be controlled it could possibly cause death by producing excessive pressure in the head. Severe swelling after an injury can press on and severely damage the spinal cord or brain. The cerebrospinal fluid (CSF) helps to clean and nourish the brain and spinal cord.

Understanding the missed lymph/brain connection is critical in helping patients with these types of injuries. Up to 48% of the CSF drains to the lymphatics. Circulation and the ability of the lymphatic system to remove excess fluid, fibrin and cellular debris out of the brain or spinal cord is especially important at the time of injury and in the rehabilitation stage. If the patient is overly acidic their lymphatic system is not flowing adequately and not able to relieve the pressure from excess fluid and proteins building in the brain or spinal cord. Without proper circulation, which the lymphatic system is a critical part of, fibrosis can occur and the injuries will not heal effectively due to scarring from the buildup of proteins.

Diet is such an important part of healing. While watching a Discovery Channel show on a little girl who was hurt in a car accident I realized how not understanding the healing power of diet can actually limit how we heal. This little girl had a spinal cord injury, lost the use of her legs and was on a ventilator to breathe after the accident. In order to try get her off the ventilator she endured intense therapy to try and build her strength in her upper body and lungs. During the months of rehabilitation the child had a lot of emotional outbursts during her therapies and at home. Now that's expected after such a life altering accident, especially for a child. What I noticed was the parents would calm her outbursts and coax her to do therapy by giving her chocolate, candies, soda and at home she got to eat what ever she wanted, which was mostly what kids eat, acid foods and soda. The girl gained weight, was getting sick a lot and by the end of therapy they couldn't get her lungs working enough to allow her to breathe without a ventilator. This meant she would probably have to be on a ventilator the rest of her life.

I believe that if the parents knew how something as simple as chocolate, candy or soda could make their daughter acidic, protein filled and limit her healing they would have given her a healthier alkaline diet. If they knew that lymphatic activation might help their daughter heal better with fewer complications they would have made sure she had lymphatic work.

World Trade Center Syndrome

Even though the toxic dust from 9/11 and the World Trade Center (WTC) has cleared, its devastation continues to hurt many of the firefighters, police, EMT's, construction workers, clean-up crews and local residents. So many are sick their illness has been named "The World Trade Center Syndrome." There are two symptoms that are most prevalent they are a chronic cough, which is so pervasive it has been dubbed the "World Trade Center Cough" and acid reflux. Other symptoms include respiratory disease, sinus problems, headaches, chronic fatigue, insomnia, muscle pain, depression, anxiety, thyroid cancer and Post Traumatic Stress Disorder. There have been 360 deaths attributed to WTC Syndrome to date, the number unfortunately is growing.

In x-rays of those with respiratory disease they are finding granulomatous pulmonary disease, swirling marks left on the lungs from foreign matter like dust. These inflammatory diseases include pulmonary fibrosis and sarcoidosis, which can be set off when exposure to dust causes the body's immune system to attack it self. The NYC Fire Department has been tracking a growing number of cases of sarcoidosis, a lung scarring disease. Typically sarcoidosis is mostly seen in the lungs but its scarring can affect any tissue or organ in the body. This growing problem is not only affecting 9/11 responders and residents who lived or worked around the WTC sight. A third of the volunteers from the WTC site came from every state and more than a dozen countries. Officials have acknowledged they are only beginning to understand the immensity of the problem. Many of these individuals are dying prematurely from fibrosis and lung disease due to a malfunctioning lymphatic system.

Let's take a look at the WTC Syndrome understanding the lymphatic system and acid-alkaline balance. As the towers collapsed concrete, glass, asbestos, dioxin, mercury, combustible materials and other debris became pulverized to a microscopic toxic dust. These tiny foreign particles entered the mouth, nostrils, eyes, and was dispersed throughout the body, especially the lungs. After many weeks and months of searching in the rubble and dust, living or working in the area, the toxic alkaline dust consisting of pulverized concrete constricted the lymphatic system, which congested and began to irritate the tissues and organs. Part of the body's healing mechanism is to produce fibrin, a protein that resembles pieces of yarn, to repair wounds or damage in the body. Fibrin is produced in the blood; it combines with blood platelets, minerals, lipids and other cellular debris to form a mesh over any damage in the tissues. Fibrosis occurs when the lymphatic system is compromised allowing an excessive amount of fibrin to accumulate in your skin, organs, bones and brain limiting circulation and tissue or organ health. Fibrosis creates limited circulation that allows acid waste to build in the tissues. The acid waste building in the tissues is what is perceived as the body's immune system attacking itself.

Those affected by the WTC dust didn't get one type of disease from their exposure. Many of the health problems that are affecting those with the WTC Syndrome affect the general population in great numbers. This book explains how a malfunctioning lymphatic system can allow proteins to build in any part of the body beginning the disease process. Remember Amyloidosis, a fatal buildup of protein in any part of the body. In the general population illnesses take time to manifest as the body slowly becomes filled with low levels of dust, acidic waste and excess proteins like fibrin and cellular debris.

At the World Trade Center site many were exposed to a massive amount of toxic dust that most of us will never see in our lifetime. With the addition of intense stress, dehydration and an overly acidic internal body their lymphatic system becomes overwhelmed, which negatively affected all systems of the body, especially the lungs. The lungs play a major role in helping to remove acid from the body. As the lymph vessels in the lungs became congested from the dust, the lung tissue itself becomes more acidic and constricts. This tightening limits circulation in the organ, allowing cellular debris and fibrin to become trapped in the tissues of the organ. This can happen in the lung or any organ limiting its function.

Those with the WTC Syndrome can finally address the true cause of their illness; a congested lymphatic system due to toxic dust overload. A congested lymphatic and circulatory system creates acidity and excess proteins in the body. The excess proteins in the body are the scarring we see in fibrosis and sclerosis that limit tissue or organ function. As with most diseases the goal is to balance the internal body and manually activate the lymphatics to help the body detox acid waste and excess proteins that are limiting your circulation and health.

Post Traumatic Stress Disorder (PTSD)

There are many names for the emotional trauma that scars veterans of war, shell shock, battle fatigue, traumatic war neurosis and now post traumatic stress disorder. Studies as far back as World War II and continuing today with the Iraq War show that large numbers of veterans return home to nightmares, sleeplessness, flashbacks, negative imagery, long term fear, depression, suicidal thoughts, aggressiveness, problems with concentration, weeping, generalized anxiety, and distress caused by recalling the battle. PTSD is an anxiety disorder that can develop after an occurrence of extreme psychological stress, such as that found in war or from a violent attack, childhood abuse, sexual abuse, or serious life threatening accident.

The lymph/ brain connection where 48% of cerebrospinal fluid (CSF) is absorbed by the lymphatics is key to understanding PTSD. When you have experienced a severe emotional trauma the body becomes overly acidic the lymphatic system congests allowing proteins and acidic waste to build in the CSF and brain. The resulting toxicity in the brain leads to many of the symptoms associated with PTSD.

In 1999 Dr. John Upledger, developer of CranioSacral Therapy and a team of therapists led 22 Vietnam veterans in a groundbreaking study which was co-designed with the West Palm Beach Veterans Administration Medical Center. In the study the Veterans received sessions of CranioSacral Therapy. An independent licensed psychologist confirmed in a post-program report that the veterans experienced fewer symptoms by the end of the program, most notably related to depression, lack of motivation, obsessive/compulsive behaviors, feelings of alienation, and total number and severity of general symptoms. More than a 95% correlation was noted between the CranioSacral Therapy sessions and the improvements the veterans saw. In CranioSacral Therapy we increase circulation in the body and membranes that surround the brain and spinal cord. The increase in cerebrospinal fluid absorption helps to calm the mind by removing acid waste and excess proteins.

Hypo or Hyperthyroid

Tens of millions of people suffer with thyroid conditions. Some of the symptoms are depression, fatigue, nervousness, weight gain or loss, muscle weakness, hair loss, difficulty concentrating and poor memory. Again, these are also signs of over acidity. The thyroid gland is located in the base of the neck above the major lymph drain. The thyroid is the closest gland to the main lymph drain, if the drain becomes congested it can lead to a backup of acid waste and proteins in the thyroid gland. The hormones it produces control cellular metabolism, or the way that cells in the body use energy.

According to Frederick P. Millard's book "Applied Anatomy of the Lymphatics" written in 1922, the thyroid is one of the most lymph involved organs in the body. If we are acidic, the circulation in the thyroid is affected, proteins build in the organ and it can't work (hypothyroid) or works too much (hyperthyroid). When I map the lymph flow to the thyroid, it is often flowing incorrectly backwards into the organ, which can congest it. Many of those with WTC Syndrome have thyroid cancer.

Arthritis

Arthritis is a circulation problem resulting in a buildup of excess proteins and acidic waste. In arthritis the circulation to your joints is impeded and the bones become acidic, toxic, protein filled and inflamed. The calcification seen on x-rays is actually protein buildup, waste and minerals that are filling the area.

Allergies

When your lymphatic system is not functioning optimally, the body becomes overwhelmed with excess waste, allergens, debris like cat dander (old cells), dust or pollen in the air and you have an allergic reaction. Our ideas of allergy testing may have to be reevaluated after looking at this new information. Healthy foods that alkalize and increase circulation can exhibit an allergic reaction by releasing stored acidic waste, proteins and toxins.

Eczema, Hives and Rashes

These conditions of the skin are irritating and sometimes painful. Eczema is a very acidic and protein congested superficial lymphatic system. The lymphatic system cleans the tissues of the body. If your superficial lymphatic system is impeded or toxic your skin may have occasional hives or become red when touched. With eczema the superficial lymphatic system is severely overly acidic and the cells and tissues are being damaged. Specific lymphatic or detox work in the start of treatment will create a severe skin irritation, the healing crisis. If you have eczema, start a detox very slowly, with extra water, nutritional supplements, especially coconut oil or fish oil supplements. Then try a few CranioSacral Therapy or massages about a week apart. Make sure you are drinking extra water and helping to move waste out of your tissues with exercise and deep breathing. As your tissues become less toxic, try Lymph Drainage Therapy or Lymphatic Cellular Detox Massage to further clean and balance your tissues. Eczema may become worse at first, as you begin to move waste out of the skin. Be sure to alkalize and balance your internal body.

During one of my lectures I met a woman and her niece who was in her thirties, confined to a wheelchair and had severe cognitive problems. The aunt explained how the niece had a bad case of eczema for over a year and that they have had a very difficult time trying to help it heal. They had just had her pH tested at her health care practitioner's office and they were told she was too alkaline. This is why just reading a test strip is dangerous. You need to understand acid-alkaline balance and the role of the lymphatic system as a sewage treatment plant. Acidic waste and proteins were storing in the arms and not making it into the urine or saliva. The niece had many large, red, inflamed, scabbed areas on her arms, that looked painful. This type of inflammation is directly related to excess acid and proteins limiting circulation in the skin

Cellulite

There are many so-called treatments for cellulite, from lasers, deep massaging machines and expensive reducing creams. Cellulite is congested tissue where lymph flow has been slowed or stopped. Fluid, proteins, fats, and metabolic waste congest the tissue creating the dimpled appearance. The only way to address the problem is to first increase lymph flow in the whole body. Then you can work on the cellulite with gentle specific Lymph Drainage Therapy (LDT) fibrotic techniques to open the congestion. It takes many sessions, but LDT is very effective at opening circulation and reducing cellulite. However, be aware that when you treat cellulite too heavily or aggressively you can damage the tissues and create saggy skin.

Incontinence and Inability to Urinate

Many people, both young and old, have a problem with the ability to hold urine. This is an acid problem. To be more specific, it is an acidic bladder problem. When your bladder, which is like a half inflated balloon, becomes acidic, it constricts and no longer has the ability to stretch easily. So instead of a balloon that can fill and collapse as necessary, the bladder becomes a tight balloon that will not give. The bladder is unable to expand when necessary and as a result, it leaks as more fluid enters the constricted bladder, this is urinary incontinence.

With urination problems, the urethra can become overly acidic, constricted and release only a trickle of urine instead of a stream of urine. Often to correct a constricted urethra it is physically stretched open in surgery, which may cause more scarring and tissue damage due to forcibly opening the tissues. This is a common problem in seniors and children. Alkalizing, hydration, removing proteins and improving circulation is an important step in addressing these problems.

Erectile Dysfunction (ED)

Erectile Dysfunction is a common, well kept secret among men. Viagra being one of the top selling drugs on the market proves it. In 2004 U.S.

sales of Viagra hit $1.1 billion. Global sales were $1.87 billion. Worldwide approximately 23 million men have tried Viagra. To make an erection it takes blood flow. If you are dehydrated, acidic or protein filled your circulation and blood volume can be affected. The tissues of the penis become constricted and there may not be enough fluid/blood in your system to allow an erection.

Studies of Viagra patients show a small number of its users are reporting vision problems. These problems can be a worsening of their vision or even a loss of peripheral vision, allowing them to see only straight ahead, as if in a tunnel. They say the vision loss is being caused by blood vessels in the eye which have become choked off as in a stroke. The cells in the choked off area may become damaged and die due to excess proteins and lack of circulation. Viagra may be stealing the blood from your extremities, especially your eyes, in order to have enough blood volume for an erection.

Infertility

My wife and I are very familiar with infertility. We tried to conceive for thirteen years. We tried almost everything but nothing worked. Sperm count can range from a low of 20 million per millimeter to 150 million per millimeter. My initial sperm count when we started to see infertility specialist's early in our marriage was 50 million sperm per millimeter. A few years later my count was down to 40 million. When we tried to conceive in our 40's I took supplements for two months to alkalize my system. The healthier cellular environment helped boost my sperm production. When we conceived our daughter, with the help of a fertility specialist, my sperm count was 150 million per millimeter.

Infertility is a silent epidemic that has few known causes. Once you understand that you may be very acidic and protein filled you will better understand when a doctor says to a woman "your body is attacking the sperm." They say it may be an autoimmune response. Sperm can't survive in an overly acidic environment. A fertilized embryo can't thrive in an overly acidic environment; this may be a cause of miscarriages. Most importantly the ovary may be filled with proteins and debris clogging the organ and limiting its ability to produce eggs. One therapist that I met had her ovaries surgically cleaned after having problems conceiving; she went on to have twins. When you are overly acidic you are filled with excess waste. A few series of sessions to activate your lymphatics starting a few months before trying to conceive, a healthy diet and nutritional support would be beneficial and help prepare both partners for their task of trying to have a baby.

Postpartum Depression

This really is a chemical imbalance in the brain caused by over acidity and a malfunctioning lymphatic system. The lymphatics help to reabsorb up to 48% of cerebrospinal fluid. A toxic or sedentary mother may be congested with excess waste from herself and the fetus in the last few weeks of pregnancy. After the birth the mother may be stressed, dehydrated and not eating or sleeping correctly. Toxicity in the mother continues to build. I saw something similar happen over and over again in my saliva pH/detoxification study. As toxicity rose, due to lymphatic activation, many participants told me they felt depressed. One even said she felt her worst depression for a day after her first lymphatic activation session.

Alopecia, Balding and Thinning Hair

Hair loss affects men and woman and is thought to be a hormonal problem. When the tiny lymph vessels in the center of the top of the head, become congested, hormones and acidic waste can build in the scalp and damage the hair follicle. When you lose part or all of the hair on your body it is called alopecia. When I have seen people with alopecia there skin appears puffy, congested. This may be caused by a stagnant and acidic superficial lymphatic system that is unable to remove excess fluid and acidic waste from the skin. Before finding out about acidosis, I was always cleaning a lot of hair from the drain after I showered and I would get dime and nickel sized bald spots in my beard. After addressing my acidosis and limited circulation my hair is staying on my head instead of in my drain and I no longer get bald spots in my beard.

Meningitis

Meningitis is an inflammation of the protective membranes that surround the brain and spinal cord, called the meninges. Meningitis may begin from viruses or bacteria, physical injury, certain medications and cancer. Some forms of meningitis are mild and end on their own, untreated meningitis can be a potentially life-threatening condition due to the closeness of the inflammation to the brain and spinal cord. The meninges are comprised of three layers of membrane that surround and protect the brain and spinal cord. Two of those layers, the dura and pia mater have lymphatic vessels. We have to look beyond the disease of meningitis and look at its root cause, stagnant and toxic fluid that leads to inflammation in the membranes that surround the brain and spinal cord. Whether from trauma, dehydration, an overly acidic diet or excess proteins the inflammation begins with limited lymph flow in the layers of the meninges.

Repetitive Stress Injuries

Repetitive stress injuries like carpal tunnel syndrome, tennis elbow, rotator cuff problems or frozen shoulder are very common. They can affect the weekend warrior who sits most of the week and then plays sports on the weekend and those that sit in front of computers typing for long periods. The excess acid can also affect a seasoned pro, like a singer who has to cancel a show because of irritated or damaged vocal cords. When you use a part of your body such as the muscles around the elbows, knees, shoulders or vocal cords they produce acidic waste. If you happened to be acidic, your lymphatic system would not pick up this waste efficiently and the buildup of toxicity would irritate and damage the tissues, especially the ligaments and tendons. This stagnant acidic waste can constrict the tissues, limit circulation and create inflammation or pain. Frozen shoulder, adhesive capsulitis, is the result of inflammation, scarring, thickening, and constricting of the capsule that surrounds the normal shoulder joint. Warm up before and stretch after physical activities to help remove acidic waste.

Ingrown Nails

Ingrown nails or its more accurate name onychocryptosis are painful inflamed nail beds that are a form of nail disease that affects millions. Even though the problem can occur in finger nails it is more prevalent in toe nails. The nail cuts into the skin creating inflammation in the nail bed. The true cause of ingrown nails is tissue acidosis. Your nail is made up of a tough protein called keratin. If the tissues around the nail were overly acidic the nail would begin to curl into the skin and create limited circulation and inflammation around the cuticle of the nail. As a young boy I would get ingrown toe nails and my mother would have to put pieces of cotton under my nails to keep the nail up out of the nail bed. As an adult I had the sides of my big toe nails removed because of recurring ingrown toe nails.

I have seen many people who have their toe nails removed because of recurring infections. The acidic and toxic environment that is curling your toenails is also causing your toenail fungus. To eliminate nail problems balance your internal body and activate the lymphatics and circulation to the toes. While on vacation my daughter started to get an ingrown nail that hurt as she walked. On vacation we don't eat as perfect as we should so I know my daughter was overly acidic. That night I activated her lymphatic system from her clavicles to her toe two or three times and by morning her pain and problem were gone and the problem hasn't occurred again. Our health problems are due to lack of circulation.

Missed Root Cause of Disease

The basis of most disease is tissue acidosis and a malfunctioning lymphatic system that allows proteins (cellular waste, fibrin) to build in the body. There are many health problems that are caused by acidosis and protein buildup which are affecting us in great numbers, i.e., heart disease, kidney disease, diabetes, Alzheimer's, lung disease, arthritis, restless leg syndrome, blood clots, polyps, fungal infections, endometriosis, cataracts and stomach aches.

The Missed Root Cause of Disease is an Undetected Acid-Alkaline Imbalance and a Malfunctioning Lymphatic System that Leads to Protein Proliferation and Limited Circulation in the Tissues and Organs of the Body.

Some Medications That Seem To Be Counter Productive

Medications are a large part of our culture. They are necessary in emergency situations or to save a life. You shouldn't be on them for your whole life when lifestyle changes may eliminate or control your disease.

Diuretics

Never Discontinue a Diuretic, Blood Thinner or any prescribed medication Without Consulting Your Doctor. It May Endanger Your Life.

When you swell, you have a lymphatic problem. Your tissues are not only accumulating water, they are accumulating large proteins. These proteins, through colloid osmotic pressure, draw water to themselves. Osmotic pressure in the circulatory system is a form of pressure exerted by proteins in blood plasma that normally tends to pull water into the circulatory system. So as diuretics remove water, some large proteins are left behind to accumulate and draw more water into your tissues, a vicious cycle.

A few times while on a long walk I ran out of water. As I began to feel dehydrated my hands and feet began to feel very tight and swollen. Many people, especially seniors, are in a constant state of dehydration. Some drink as little as a cup of water a day because they don't want to be running to the bathroom. They are self-limiting their water intake, which creates more problems. Without water your body becomes acidic and fluid, wastes and proteins collect in the tissues. Individuals who have a problem with mild swelling feel an immediate relief in their tight and congested limbs after the first session of lymph drainage therapy. Lymphatic activation, balancing the body and learning ways to help reduce excess proteins help to control swelling.

Decongestants and Antihistamines

The adult body is between 60%-70% water. Your blood is just over 90% water. Your lymph is 96% water and your cerebrospinal fluid is 98.5% water. Your health is dependent on a well hydrated body.

When you take decongestants or antihistamines you are dehydrating your body. The medication may alleviate your symptoms, but by being dehydrated your blood and body become concentrated with more waste and toxins. This waste will eventually bring on another allergy attack or sinus infection. Dehydration limits lymphatic flow, circulation and the removal of waste and allergens from the body.

Rat Poison as a Blood Thinner

As you age, your blood becomes thick from the accumulating wastes, cellular debris and escaped proteins. The blood can actually become the consistency of ketchup. This can further impede circulation through your tissues causing blood clots, heart attacks or strokes.

Warfarin, also called Coumadin, is a blood thinner that interferes with the body's ability to recycle vitamin K. It is creating a shortage of vitamin K in your body that can lead to a life-threatening deficiency. Many of today's popular products to kill rodents work by creating a vitamin K deficiency. If severe enough it leads to the animal bleeding to death.

A question that needs to be answered is, why are we filling with waste in the first place? The answer is a toxic tissue acidosis that interferes with the ability of the lymphatic system to clean our tissues. Lymphatic Cellular Detox Massage, CranioSacral Therapy or Lymph Drainage Therapy all help to remove waste, excess fluids and proteins. This changes the pH level of the body, allowing the lymphatic system to then do its job of keeping us clean of waste. Fruits, vegetables, being hydrated, exercise and systemic enzymes are a safer and healthier alternative to blood thinners. Never stop a blood thinner without consulting your physician.

Coumadin as a life saving drug may be necessary but we shouldn't be living on it for decades. There are better and more beneficial ways to make your blood flow, such as a greener diet, hydrating and alkalizing your body, lymphatic activation and taking systemic enzymes. Consult with a health care practitioner who is familiar with thinning your blood using systemic enzymes.

Cholesterol Lowering Medications

Your lymphatic system helps remove cholesterol and triglycerides from your tissues. When you are acidic your lymphatic system is impeded and lipids and fat can become trapped in the tissues and accumulate. Your body needs cholesterol. It is a necessary component of every cell and is vital to the cells structure and function. Instead of using medications to lower cholesterol, try the 80/20 diet, exercise and other ideas in this book to alkalize and increase your lymph flow in order to drain cholesterol from your tissues.

Health Promoting Basics

The key to most of your health problems becomes simple if you understand the acid-alkaline theory and its affect on the lymphatic system. The basis of disease is stagnant, overly acidic and protein rich fluid in your tissues, i.e. skin, muscles, bones, organs and central nervous system. If you have a health problem you need to alkalize to create a healthier inner environment. Then increase lymph flow and blood circulation so oxygen and nutrients can move throughout your body, and waste can be eliminated from your tissues.

Start with two sessions of massage, CranioSacral Therapy or Lymph Drainage Therapy a week apart. Begin doing some mild exercise to increase circulation to move oxygen and extra nutrition to the cells. Create a healthier cellular environment in your tissues by eating a 90% alkaline diet, take a multivitamin supplement (more than the RDA), as well as alkalizing supplements and systemic enzymes. These protein lysing (eating) enzymes help remove trapped excess protein that may be limiting your circulation, as in fibrosis or scar tissue from an injury or surgery. Drink mineralized water often throughout the day especially before meals and at bedtime. Obtain a series of lymphatic activations after you have started greening your diet and are taking nutritional supplements. You will feel less of a detox reaction if you have alkaline minerals in your body to neutralize excess acid that may be produced by the lymphatic activation. Start Self-Lymphatic Activation slowly, once every few days then gently self-activate your lymphatic system on a daily basis.

If you are very sick, do a detox slowly under a doctor's supervision. Try meditating with deep breathing at least three times a day to increase circulation to the body and affected area. Even just 3-5 minutes three times a day can make a difference. Always take two deep breaths together every few minutes. Now you have taken control of the situation and are taking proactive steps to help change the disease process.

Detox Baths are Convenient

The idea of soaking in mineral rich waters to improve health has been used for thousands of years. It makes sense. We know that more and more medications like nicotine or nitroglycerin patches or medications for ADHD are now being made in skin patches to be absorbed right through the skin. Mineral baths are an easy way to help your body become more alkaline. You can go to a spa that has mineral baths or you can have a similar experience by soaking at home in an Epsom salt bath (magnesium sulfate). It is a very easy and inexpensive way to relax or detox the body.

When you take a warm Epsom salt bath you are helping to open your lymph flow and blood circulation by alkalizing and warming the tissues of the body. When adding the Epsom salt to your bath, add three big handfuls. If you want to use an Epsom salt bath to relax, take a fifteen to thirty minute soak, making sure to drink water and incorporate some deep breathing. When you are in the bath be sure to go low enough into the water so that the water touches just below your chin for periods of time. This is important because you want to make sure the water has a chance to contact the main drain by the clavicles. Taking a mineral bath occasionally can help to destress you, taking a few baths on consecutive days can help to detox and balance your body.

I use Epsom salt baths for myself and my family to help detox acid waste from our body's. If I am doing an Epsom salt bath on a few consecutive days, I will eat lighter, include more water, exercise and do some self-lymphatic activation. Often after the third day I feel tight, have a headache and feel excess acid rising up my esophagus into my throat. The next day it is gone and I feel better, healthier. Never take three baths to start out because it will congest and overwhelm your body. If you have any health concerns first consult with your health care practitioner.

When you want to concentrate on a specific type of detoxification bath you must look at LL's Magnetic Clay Detox Baths. This company has been in business since 1995 preparing clay baths with spices and herbs for natural detoxification for use in the privacy of your own home. They have specific clay formulas to help detox mercury, environmental toxins, formaldehyde, aluminum, cadmium from smoking, lead and copper. These clay baths are simple but powerful. If you are sick, start slowly for only a few minutes to avoid a severe detox reaction. Be well hydrated and replace minerals that may be lost during the detox bath. This is a great product to help detox children and adults.

CHAPTER TWELVE

Syndromes of Uncertain Origin

A Silent Killer

When you look at page 2480 of the seventeenth edition of the Merck Manual (a physician's reference), you will see a section called "Syndromes of Uncertain Origin." In the opening paragraph it mentions how many of us suffer from syndromes for which no cause can be found. It also mentions how these syndromes are often seen as having psychologic causes, meaning "it's in your head."

I have had patients who have experienced this. We are missing how acid and a malfunctioning lymphatic system can silently tighten your tissues or affect your brain. Excess acid waste is not seen as the culprit, so it is overlooked or seen as a digestive inconvenience. The important fact is that after I increased their lymph flow, within a few sessions these patients felt better and had less of their symptoms, or their problem went away entirely. So it's not in their head. When we look at these Syndromes of Uncertain Origin, and include an acidic pH and a malfunctioning lymphatic system, an origin becomes more evident.

Gulf War Syndrome

The Gulf War Syndrome has affected 5,000 to 80,000 U.S. veterans (from 1991). Now that we are fighting a war in Iraq, in the next few years we may see many more soldiers with this unexplained syndrome. Some of the symptoms these soldiers have suffered with are chronic fatigue, skin rashes, unexplained hair loss, headaches, muscle pain, numbness in the extremities, loss of memory, problems thinking, nervous system disorders, problems with their respiratory systems, sleep problems, cardiovascular problems, menstrual problems, diarrhea or constipation. All of these problems are also symptoms of over acidity and can be caused by many of the military scenarios these soldiers experienced. Having been in the military for three years in the late 1970's and understanding acidosis and the lymphatic system, I can easily see how these soldiers could have been made extremely toxic by their military service in the Gulf area. In the next few sections I will explain how I believe the military diet, repeated, intense stress, heat, dehydration, many vaccinations, experimental drugs to protect the soldiers against nerve gas, insect repellents, pesticides, and possibly small doses of nerve gas and other chemical weapons that may have been in the air, could have made these soldiers very toxic which may be leading to their current health problems. Many circumstances add up together to create illness.

Military Diet

The military does not skimp on feeding their soldiers. If they are eating in a mess hall there is a variety of foods to choose from including fruits and vegetables. If given choices of what to eat, even though there may be alkaline foods, most of the young soldiers eat meat, chicken, pasta, breads and desserts. The majority of the food served and eaten is acid forming. When I served in the Army, for breakfast we would have eggs, pancakes, sausage, bacon, white toast, numerous cups of coffee and orange juice. Lunch would be a choice of fried chicken, beef, meat sandwiches, hamburger, fries, coffee, soda or iced tea and dessert. Dinner would be beef, chicken, fish, rice or pasta, coffee, soda or iced tea, ice cream or cake. Vegetables were always available, but very few soldiers took them. If we were in the field on maneuvers, the c-rations, now called MRE's (meals ready to eat) were all acid. Most of the time the MRE's were canned beef, peanut butter, white crackers, hot cocoa and chocolate. In the military there is always plenty of coffee to drink throughout the day. The military diet is very acid forming.

Intense Stress

War is very stressful, even for soldiers who are well trained for war. In the Gulf War, the use of chemical weapons was always a threat. The soldiers knew that Saddam Hussein had used them on his own people, so the possibility of a chemical attack was always imminent. Anytime there was a threat of chemical weapons or a scud missile attack the soldiers had to don protective suits and masks. The threats were daily and often. These soldiers were donning their protective gear various times during the day and night. Stress immediately reduces your circulation and is very acid forming to your body. Repeated and prolonged stress can be deadly.

During my time in the military, during a peace time era, I experienced a small sample of this stress during war maneuvers in Germany. This is similar to playing war and in an effort to make it realistic they would set off tear gas canisters around our vehicles. I can tell you first hand that when we received an alert that gas was in the area, your stress level intensified and your heart would race while donning your protective gear. This was only simulating war; I can only imagine what it must have been like for these soldiers, under the real threat of attack over and over again.

Heat and Dehydration

Living in Arizona I can tell you when it's 110 degrees out the sweat doesn't even have time to form on your body. The air is pulling moisture from your body and dehydration can occur quickly. During the Gulf War in the dry season, it was often over 115 degrees. Heat and dehydration are very acid forming to the body. The lymphatic system is over 90% water and is responsible for cleaning the tissues. When we are dehydrated the lymphatic system cannot work efficiently, leaving proteins and waste in the tissues and organs.

Neurotoxins

Many toxins can affect your nervous system. Soldiers are exposed to many toxins, especially during war. Beginning with the many vaccinations they receive in order to travel overseas, including the experimental pyridostigmine bromide, an anti-nerve gas drug. They may have also been exposed to neurotoxins such as the nerve gas sarin, insect repellents, pesticides, fumes from oil fires and chemical weapons such as depleted uranium. All of these toxins, (many of which produce Dioxin) an overly acidic diet, intense repeated stress and dehydration can make the soldiers very toxic, overly acidic and impair their lymphatic system which can affect any system in the body.

Depleted Uranium

According to one retired Gulf War doctor, many of the soldiers are suffering with kidney problems and other diseases from the higher than normal levels of depleted uranium. The uranium is coated onto shells to help them penetrate heavy tank armor. Once it explodes, the depleted uranium particles become part of the air around the soldiers, entering into their lungs. Depleted uranium can cause cancer and other health problems. In the 1991, Gulf War experts estimate over 320 tons of depleted uranium were exploded.

I recently met a Gulf War Vet who told me of a letter he recently received from the Secretary of Defense. The letter was warning him that soldiers that were in his battalion are experiencing much higher than normal rates of brain cancer compared to other soldiers in the Gulf War. Some members of his battalion had the unfortunate responsibility of exploding captured or unexploded munitions. Many of these munitions contained depleted uranium. He told me that after the war, he was very violent, aggressive and would have bouts of depression. For the last few years his lymph nodes swell often for no reason. Our veterans need help. Balancing the body and lymphatic activation may play an important role in helping these vets clean their toxic bodies.

One Internet site I viewed was trying to debunk the Gulf War Syndrome. They associated the soldiers' symptoms to the mysterious disease called Multiple Chemical Sensitivity Syndrome. Most doctors think that this syndrome has psychological causes and is not a real illness. They are wrong. When we become toxic the lymphatic system becomes overwhelmed and limits how our organs and brain function. These soldiers were negatively affected by their military experience.

Iraq War

The Iraq War was not mentioned in the chapter on "Symptoms of Unknown Origin." According to researchers at the University of California, San Francisco nearly one third of the Iraq, Afghanistan veterans are returning home with mental health problems like depression, anxiety and post traumatic stress disorder. The major difference between the Gulf War vets and those in Afghanistan and Iraq is the duration of time spent in combat. Since the mission in Iraq and Afghanistan has lasted many years, many of the vets have been called back to serve in these combat regions 2 and 3 times. Ongoing relentless stress constricts the lymphatic system negatively affecting the organs and central nervous system creating depression, PTSD or negative thoughts like suicide. Many of these veterans are on multiple antidepressant medications. The rate of suicide attempts among vets is escalating quickly. It is hard to get an accurate number from the Veterans Affairs but it has been reported that over 1000 vets a month are trying to take their own life. Medications are not the answer. Many of these vets are on multiple medications for their stress and depression.

Traumatic brain injury is another area where understanding the lymphatic system and its connection to the CSF and brain could help these vets. Many vets are coming home with brain injuries due to exploding IED's. In brain injuries fibrosis can occur limiting circulation of cerebrospinal fluid and healing. Balancing the body and activating the lymphatic system would help improve their ability to heal and think clearly. Many Iraq veterans are coming home as amputees. Understanding the lymphatic system could help those vets that have lost limbs have less stress, anxiety, swelling and pain after their surgery and during recovery.

Multiple Chemical Sensitivity Syndrome (MCS)

There are toxic chemicals and allergens in the air, water and in the food you eat. Many chemicals have the ability to make your body toxic by compromising your lymphatic system. With a person who already has a compromised immune system, one exposure to a toxic chemical or allergen can make them very ill by seriously impairing their lymphatic system and circulation further. When the lymphatic system is seriously impaired, acidic waste, proteins and toxins can build in your tissues and organs. With repeated exposure, at some point the system is overloaded, shuts down and becomes severely toxic. Some known reported triggers for MCS are fumes from paint, carpet and furniture odors, alcohol, drugs, caffeine, food additives, fuel odors, engine exhaust, perfumes, pesticides and herbicides. These triggers also add to the acidity of the body by negatively affecting the lymphatic system. Symptoms of MCS include fatigue, a rapid heart rate, chest pain, coughing, shortness of breath, flushing, sweating, dizziness, nausea, choking, hoarseness, trembling, numbness, and difficulty concentrating. Again, most of these are signs of acidosis.

Chronic Fatigue Syndrome

Chronic fatigue syndrome is not your everyday fatigue. It is severely debilitating. Very often people can no longer function in their regular daily life. This may last for months or years. The Merck Manual says the symptoms are made worse by exercise, any exertion, sore throat, headache and other stresses. When those with chronic fatigue exert themselves, exercise, or are stressed, they have to deal with excess acidic waste, proteins and toxins in their system creating a healing crisis. This is a worsening of their symptoms, a flare-up. Besides fatigue, some symptoms are headaches, weakness, tend
and joint aches, insomnia and an inability to concentr
signs of acidosis.

In writing this book I have noticed that mar
many of the same symptoms, especially fatigue and i
ity to think. Knowing about the lymph/brain connec
ther validates that many of our diseases involve acidos

lymphatic system. Acidosis and excess proteins impairs the ability of the red blood cells to circulate and carry oxygen to the cells. Without oxygen your cells cannot make energy. You need to balance your body, move your blood and breathe deeply to create energy and think clearly.

Proper Maintenance

Do you remember the last time you took the time to thoroughly clean your internal body to improve your physical and mental wellbeing? If you didn't clean your house A/C filter, the A/C would breakdown. Your body works the same way, it needs to be cleaned a few times a year to lose weight and have health. In the next few chapters you will learn five basic steps that will help you balance your body, activate your lymphatic system and promote optimal heal.

5 Steps to Balance, Activate the Lymph and Optimal Health

The Goal

In the next 15-30 days the goal is to incorporate the 5 Steps into your life. Begin by making small lifestyle changes to gently detox and balance the internal body, to optimize lymphatic function and health.

1- Learn Your Warning Signs Of Toxicity
When you become out of balance for an extended period of time you experience symptoms like tight muscles, headaches, gas, bloating, acid reflux, IBS, thinning hair and insomnia are all signs of a toxic body. You become affected where you have least circulation. Being aware of your signs of toxicity is key.

2- Green-Up Your Diet "80/20 Rule."
Eat significantly more fruits and vegetables. Supplement your diet.

3- Increase Your Circulation:
Exercise, Deep Breathing, Hydration and Posture
Health begins with daily exercise, taking two very deep breaths every few minutes, drinking adequate amounts of mineralized water and good posture.

- Stress Reduction
ss is severely acid forming; it can negatively affect your whole body in a
conds.

Detoxification – The Real Key to Optimal Health
ivation or Self-Lymphatic Activation

CHAPTER THIRTEEN

Step One: Learn the Warning Signs of Toxicity

Tight Muscles are Overly Acidic Tissues

Most of you go through life with tight muscles, especially in your neck, shoulders and low back. It is very important to realize that when you are tight you are acidic and toxic. Tight muscles mean your cellular environment is overly acidic, making the cells, tissues, muscles and vessels constrict from the toxicity. I asked a few of my patients who have migraines if they can tell when they are about to get a migraine. Most of them said they feel the muscles in their neck or shoulders tighten and become sore prior to their migraines. This is an important sign! When you feel muscles tighten you should get a massage or lymphatic activation session. You should also balance your body by drinking more water, eat a greener diet or fast for a few days to stop the oncoming migraine. Your health is in your own hands. Watch for your specific signs of toxicity.

Physical Signs of Toxicity

Instead of just listing the signs and symptoms of acidity, I decided to list the problems I had with acid during my life. Problems that I now know were caused by an undetected tissue acidosis and its affect on my lymphatic system. Since changing my inner environment to a healthier alkaline state I no longer have these problems. They include gas, indigestion, bloating, hemorrhoids, stuttering, hair loss, warts, eczema, hives, cracks in the heels of the feet, heel pain, lactose intolerance, constipation, irritable bowel syndrome, fatigue, fluid filled cysts, weight gain, headaches, migraines, allergies, hives, thinning hair, back pain, neck pain, joint pain, swollen tongue, bone spurs, inability to use my hands, inability to think clearly, anxiety, aggressiveness, insomnia, and the inability to concentrate.

Signs of Toxicity in Children

When the tissues, muscles or organs in a child are overly acidic, they tighten and can become toxic. This toxicity can affect your children in many ways starting with colic, stomach problems, ear infections, stuttering, recurring colds, skin problems, weight problems, muscle twitches, tight back or neck, walking stiffly or walking on their toes due to acidic and contracted muscles in their lower legs. When acidosis affects the ability of their lymphatic system to drain their cerebrospinal fluid, they may have headaches, seizures, insomnia, hyperactivity, aggressiveness, anxiety, depression, compulsive disorders and problems thinking. If you ignore your child's little idiosyncrasies now, they may continue to congest into adulthood and may begin to have depression, anxiety or become bipolar.

Saliva pH Testing

We have already discussed how testing your blood for pH levels is not a good idea. Blood will take minerals from your bones and skin to keep at a constant pH of 7.37 to 7.43. Your saliva pH, as it enters the mouth from the parotid gland, is slightly acidic at 6.4 to 6.9. As the saliva loses carbon dioxide in the mouth, it becomes more alkaline and may be between 7.0 to 7.5. The parotid and submandibular glands produce saliva. Saliva pH testing is an accurate measure of the pH of the tissues and muscles above the clavicles in the neck and head. (See Fig. 13.01) As the lymph fluid drains down the face and neck to the clavicle nodes, the lymph vessels pass over and sometimes through the parotid and submandibular glands. Lymph nodes surround these glands, they can be anywhere around the glands. These glands are responsible for 80% of your saliva production. If acidic waste is building up in the tissues and lymph vessels around these glands, the saliva would reflect the change in the tissue pH. Remember most of our diseases are tissue diseases such as cancer, lupus, heart disease, arthritis, diabetes, fibromyalgia, candida, etc.

Urine pH Testing

In testing the toxicity of your tissues, testing your urine can give you significantly more information. Testing your saliva pH is only showing you the state of the tissues above your clavicles. Even though you may have good flow in your face and neck, by the glands that produce saliva, your circulation in the tissues below the clavicles in your body may be impeded and toxic. That is why we need to test both saliva and urine to understand the state of toxicity in your overall tissues. Saliva and urine pH testing, plus a medial history of the person tested, can be more conclusive. When testing urine we are measuring the

Superficial Lymph Circulation of the Neck, Face and Head

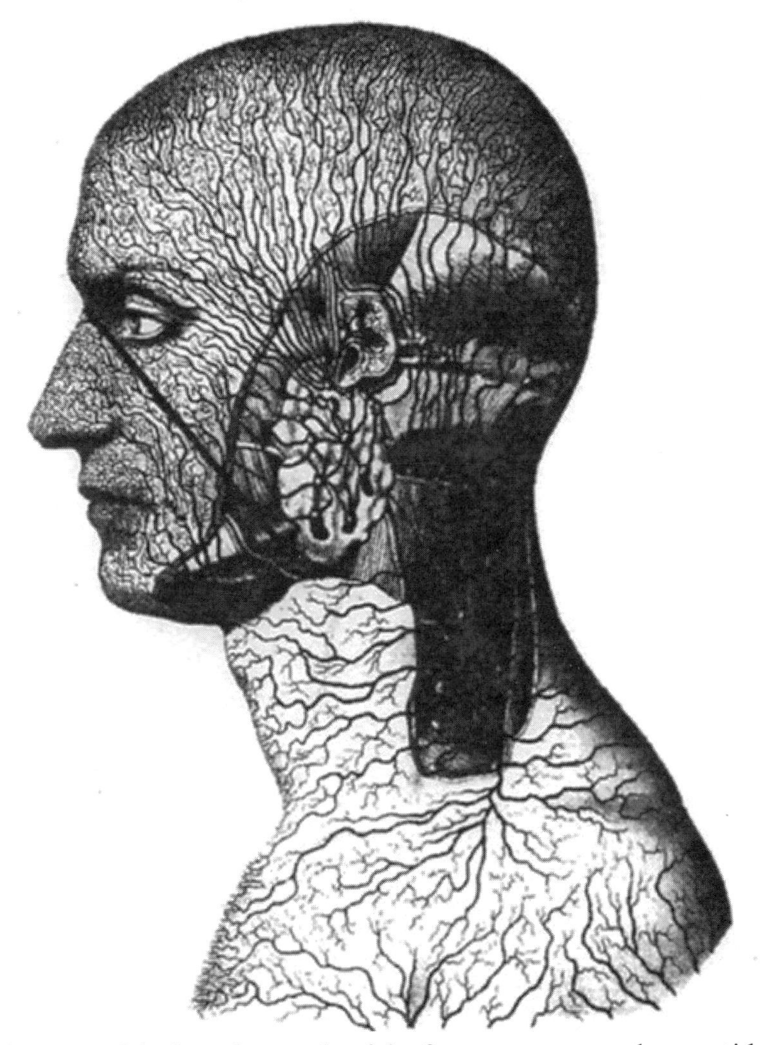

Fig. 13.01 Many of the lymph vessels of the face converge on the parotid gland below the ear. Saliva pH testing is a way to measure the acidity of these tissues and surrounding areas in the mouth.

pH level of fluid that is leaving the body. The fluid leaving the body should test more acidic if the acid wastes are actually leaving the tissues and entering the lymphatic system. If acid is leaving the body the urine pH should be below 7.0, if you are taking a few basic supplements.

You Still May be Toxic with a Healthy pH Test

According to test strip manufacturers if your pH is between 6.5-7.5, you are in a healthy pH range. That has to be clarified. I can tell you that if you follow those guidelines you may be missing that you are storing acid in your skin, muscles, bones, organs and brain. In a study collecting the data from people who self-tested their saliva and urine pH, I noticed that some individuals who had health problems had a normal urine pH between 7.0-7.5. These tests showed me that they are not perfect and cannot show if a tissue, (i.e. spleen, liver or digestive system) is acidic.

According to the pamphlets that come with pH test strips, this is within a healthy range. I believe these results need to be clarified further. If you are taking no supplements or only a multivitamin and maybe some C or E, your urine pH should be slightly acidic around 6.3-6.5. This means acid is actually leaving the body. If you test over 7.0 and aren't taking a lot of alkalizing supplements, acid may actually be storing in your tissues creating a hostile and damaging cellular environment. You will learn that anytime you feel tight, fatigued and sore or have headaches you are becoming more acidic and filled with protein.

If you test within a healthy range, but have health problems, you have to realize that you are probably toxic and storing acid waste in your tissues and organs. I have seen this many times in my studies; a patient who has many serious health concerns has normal saliva and urine pH tests. After they have a few sessions to activate their lymphatic system their pH levels first become very acidic, as acid is leaving the body and then moves more into balance.

If you test in a normal range but have health problems, recheck your pH after increasing your circulation on a couple of consecutive days to push out acid waste. There are many ways to increase your circulation exercise, massage, self-lymphatic activation, CranioSacral Therapy, Lymph Drainage Therapy, Lymphatic Cellular Detox Massage or warm Epsom salt bathes.

Don't Become Obsessed – Be Aware

When I first tested my family it really opened my eyes to acidosis. For a few weeks I was obsessed with testing them every few days. This isn't necessary. Once you test and see that you may be acidic and toxic, start following the 5 Steps to create balance and activate the lymphatics and in your body. You can then test your pH weekly or monthly. Once you see that you are becoming tight, or your problems are returning, you are becoming toxic again. Keeping your body in balance and your lymph flow moving is a constant struggle. Due to hectic lives we too often learn to ignore our tight muscles and pain until it has become a more serious problem. Being aware of how your body feels is half the battle to balancing your health.

An Exception

There is one exception that needs to be considered. That exception is whether you are taking large amounts of alkalizing supplements to buffer the excess acid. If you are taking large amounts, especially mineral rich supplements, your urine should be 7.0 to 7.5. Taking a multiple vitamin once a day or a few supplements such as vitamins A, C, or E does not equate to large amounts of supplements. In my daily routine, I take many of the products I mention in Chapter Sixteen. Testing your urine pH is very important when you take large amounts of nutritional supplements. Being too alkaline is just as damaging as being too acidic. If your urine pH is over 7.5, reduce your mineral supplementation for a few days, hydrate and exercise to move your blood and retest.

Proper pH Testing

When you buy your pH strips look for one that goes down to 5.0 or 4.5 rather than 5.5. It is important to fast from food, beverages and water for two hours before you test your saliva or urine pH. If you need water for health reasons, it may be taken up to one hour before the test. Anything you put in your mouth will alter the results. No tooth brushing, gum, mints, cigarettes or cigars for two hours before the test.

Testing Saliva pH

Testing your saliva is a good indicator of how acidic or alkaline the tissues and structures above your shoulders may be. Most of the lymph in the body converges in a vein beneath the left clavicle bone. The lymph in the neck and head must flow down to the clavicle. The lymph in the body, for the most part, flows up to the base of the neck. If your lymph flow were congested it would back up into the neck and then the head, similar to a damned river.

To collect saliva swallow a few times and collect fluid in the bottom of your mouth and transfer it into a clean spoon or container. Place the pH test strip in the saliva for a few seconds making sure the piece of paper on the strip is completely wet.

Testing Urine pH

Testing urine allows you to see the pH of the fluid that was in your kidneys and bladder as it is leaving your body. When testing after you wake in the morning, urinate and then test your second urination of the morning. Have nothing by mouth until you test your urine. Start by collecting a few ounces of urine in a container or place the pH test strip in the stream of urine for a few seconds making sure the piece of paper on the strip is completely wet.

Finding Your pH Level

If you want to attain health and prevent or overcome disease you need to understand how to read your pH test results accurately. After removing the strip from the fluid being tested let the strip sit for 20-60 seconds (depends on manufacturer). Don't wait too long to read the strip, it can dry out and the color and results will change. Compare the color of your test strip to the color on the pH chart that came with your test strips and find the closest match. You can test at any time of day, just fast for two hours before testing. pH tends to be more acidic in the morning and becomes more alkaline as the day goes on. Test your urine and saliva pH twice a day for a few days, then take an average, this will give you a more accurate view of your pH.

CHAPTER FOURTEEN

Step Two: Green-Up Your Diet, "The 80/20 Rule"

Alkaline Diet Has Many Health Benefits

Our diet is passed down from each generation, from family member to family member. Diet should be considered when family members get the same diseases. Today's American diet is overly processed and mostly acid forming foods and beverages. Our overly acidic diet is a major contributing factor in why we are extremely tired, sick or obese. Eating too many acid producing foods are very unhealthy and actually the opposite of what we should be eating, fruits and vegetables. We eat a great deal of pasta, chocolate, beef, chicken, fish, bread, eggs, rice and we drink coffee, tea, soda, beer and wine. Researchers have found evidence that as far back as Hippocrates, people were told to eat more vegetables and fruits, which are alkaline forming foods, and less meat and grains, which are acid forming foods, to rid their body of illness.

If I had been told as a child that my choices in food or drink could either kill me or heal me, I may have made different choices earlier on. Many people take the easy way out and say "I eat what my body wants or I eat what makes me happy". It may make you happy in the short term, but the long term health consequences of not understanding acid-alkaline balance are very scary; namely obesity, cancer, heart disease, diabetes, aggressive aging, and Alzheimer's. Unfortunately, eating without understanding the impact food has on your health is foolish. When you learn what foods are acid or alkaline forming in your body, you will have the right information to make better choices for a healthier, happier life.

Study Shows An Alkaline Diet Benefits Genes

According to a study in the journal Proceedings of the National Academy of Sciences comprehensive diet and lifestyle changes can create swift and dramatic changes at the genetic level. The research was led by Dr. Dean Ornish, head of the Preventative Medicine Research Institute in Sausalito, California. In a small study, 30 men with low risk prostate cancer went through three months of major lifestyle and diet changes. The men ate a diet high in alkaline fruits, vegetables, whole grains, legumes, added moderate exercise like walking a half-hour a day and an hour of stress management such as meditation. The men lost weight, lowered their blood pressure and saw other health improvements. According to the study the activity of disease-preventing genes increased while a number of disease-promoting genes, including those involved in prostate and breast cancer, shutdown. Dr. Ornish stated "It's an exciting finding because so often people say, 'Oh, it's all in my genes, what can I do?' Well, it turns out you may be able to do a lot." "In just three months, I can change hundreds of my genes simply by changing what I eat and how I live?' That's pretty exciting." Dr. Ornish a leader in his field is on the right track.

Fruits and Vegetables Lower Cholesterol

There really is a certain way we should be eating and it's not the government food pyramid, Atkins, Weight Watchers, The Zone, or most diets. We are meant to eat mostly fruits, vegetables and some whole grains which are more alkaline, and very little of everything else that is acid, like meats and processed white flour products. According to the Merck Manual, fruits and vegetables lower cholesterol. Cholesterol lowering drugs are used by tens of millions of you. Fruits and vegetables are alkaline forming in the body and improve circulation by dilating vessels which allows the lymphatic system to drain cholesterol from your tissues. Instead of taking medications to lower cholesterol that may have other consequences on your body, you should eat more fruits and vegetables.

Too Much of a Good Thing!

Food is one of my passions. It makes me very happy. I grew up in Brooklyn, New York the Mecca for food enthusiasts. Each neighborhood, whether it was Italian, Thai, Japanese, Chinese, Cuban, Jamaican, Indian or Greek, had its treasures and I knew them all. My parents were also food enthusiasts and were always opening our eyes to new cuisine. Food was an important part of our family life, everything revolved around food. I love to eat, to me it's an experience. Whether it's a Nathan's hot dog in Coney Island or an aged steak at Peter Lugers in Queens; I savor the experience. Before I learned about acidosis, my diet, even as a young boy, consisted of everything acid: meat, eggs, bread, pasta, pizza, rice, chocolate, soda, and iced tea. My family always had 2 cases of generic soda in the house. I don't remember drinking much water and I had violent stomach pains right after I ate. I always wondered why I twitched my nose (like a rabbit) continually for almost a year. Now I know I was very dehydrated. I didn't realize that it was my overly acidic diet and lifestyle choices (like drinking soda and not water) that made me toxic and sick. I was pouring too much acid into my body. As an adult if I was out to dinner I would drink beer or a pitcher of iced tea and then have some coffee or espresso after the meal. If any of you drink a lot of coffee or tea, stop wondering why you have stomach problems, tight muscles, stress, headaches and insomnia or are tired all the time. Coffee and tea are acid forming in your body.

Eat Healthy Most of the Time

Many of the books on acid-alkaline diets suggest you eat a vegetarian diet. Being a food lover, I don't believe many people will have much long-term success with this type of restrictive diet. There is too much influence from the world we live in. We are bombarded by food advertisements everywhere we turn. Instead of giving up on your favorite foods, you need to eat more alkaline foods (fruits, vegetables and some whole grains) most of the time and have a little acid food once in a while as a treat. When I say have a treat, remember you are treating yourself and your children with acid forming or protein laden foods that will limit circulation and health. Eating excess acid forming foods on a daily basis will catch up with you. The saying "we are what we eat", makes much more sense now. If we eat excessive amounts of acid foods we become out of balance, toxic and sick. Changing your life for the better is not going to be easy. You will have to make some small changes. My father would always say, "if it's easy, it's probably wrong." It has taken me almost a year to realize that I feel better when I eat healthier. So take the pressure off and know that over the next year you have a lot to learn about balance in your body. Then you will be empowered for the rest of your life. You will have the information to make better choices for health, happiness and to reclaim your life.

Get Back on the Band Wagon

My wife and I feel life is to be enjoyed and a big part of that enjoyment is socializing and eating. Knowing how to balance your acid-alkaline levels allows you to eat healthfully most of the time, especially at home. Then you can enjoy yourself with small portions of acid forming foods and beverages when you are dining out without feeling guilty. This way your diet isn't so restricted. If you have a craving for something not so healthy and you haven't had it for a while, go ahead and have it. Acknowledge that it is not a good choice, eat it, enjoy it, and immediately get back on the bandwagon and eat greener the next few meals to help balance your internal body. After a while of eating healthier, the foods we normally enjoyed don't have the same appeal, your tastes will change. Have you ever noticed that after weeks or months of dieting it doesn't take much to make you feel heavier. When I start eating more acid foods or drink, within one or two days I feel and look heavier. This is not just fat accumulating quickly, it is also fluid that is not being picked up by your lymphatic system for elimination.

The "80/20 Rule"

Once you understand which foods are alkaline or acid forming, all diets become the "80/20 Rule". This simple rule has been written about in a few acid-alkaline diet books. We need to learn to eat 80% alkaline forming foods, which are vegetables, fruits and some grains and eat 20% acid forming foods like meats, fish, eggs and grains. By the end of the day you want to be in the "80/20 Zone". When you first change your diet, especially if you are a diabetic, consume more vegetables and less fruit, until your body is more in balance. If I know I am going out to dinner or to a party where I will typically eat more acid foods or drink, I will try and limit my two other meals to fruits and vegetables. There have been times when I needed to eat fruits and vegetables for a few days to counteract the large amounts of acid producing foods and drinks I had in a weekend or at a party. Life is to be enjoyed. The key is watching and balancing your intake, you are responsible for your health. To make it simpler try making your portion of meat, chicken, fish or pasta become the side dish not the main part of your meal. Measure your portion of acid by eye. You need to eat four times the acid portion in fruits and vegetables.

An Easy Decision

The "80/20 Rule" is simple and it's the only diet tip you will ever need to know. Before I learned about acid-alkaline balance I thought I was eating a relatively healthy diet. I tried to include a few fruits and vegetables in my day, but the problem was I kept eating too many acid foods. I was probably eating 90% acid to 10% alkaline forming foods. At times I could have been eating all acid foods and consuming many iced tea's throughout the day.

Now I understand why I had tight, sore muscles and a sensitive stomach. I was continually putting acid into my body in one form or another. I was poisoning myself with what I thought were healthy foods such as pasta, beef, chicken, white bread and white rice. Once I actually understood how our everyday diet is full of acid foods and proteins that harm us, it was easier for me to make healthier decisions in eating. It hasn't been a walk in the park. The more I followed the "80/20 Rule" of eating more fruit and vegetables, the more I noticed that I felt better, no aches and pains, gas or bloating.

I give all of the credit for changing our diet to my wife, Eileen. She has made our transition to a greener diet a flavorful journey. There were many times when she said "What do I feed you?" Our diet was meat, pasta, rice and a small amount of vegetables. Now there are times you can open my refrigerator and see nothing but fruits and vegetables.

Atkins, South Beach Diet and Weight Watchers

Most people who say they were following the Atkins Diet, were taking the meat thing too literally. Excessive amounts of meat, chicken and fish are acid forming in the body and make you toxic and tight. Your cells are constricting and being damaged from the unhealthy environment. The Atkins "Low-Carb" fad is thankfully fading away. The few times I saw Dr. Atkins on television interviews his refrigerator was filled with vegetables. He would sit down to eat and his plate would be filled with salad and vegetables next to his steak. His portion looked to be 50% alkaline and 50% acid. This is better than 80% acid foods, but it is still too much acid. Eating 80% alkaline and 20% acid allows you to have a small amount of meat, pasta or an acid treat. Most people can live with eating more alkaline most of the time because it is not totally restrictive if they know it will make them healthier.

The South Beach Diet is another popular diet. I recently escorted my mother to a doctor's visit, he had just received the South Beach Diet book. He was recommending the diet to his patients who needed to lose weight. I asked him if he thought the diet allowed people to eat too many acid-forming foods. He told me that the diet is meant to make you more acidic, to burn fat. You see, we don't realize we are already too acidic.

Most of my family have lost weight and swear by Weight Watchers. Even though they have all lost weight they need to work hard to maintain their weight and most are severely acidic. Weight Watchers works on a points system, you try to keep your points at a preset number by the end of the day. Weight Watchers is on to something. They allow you to eat as many vegetables as you want for no points. As many vegetables as you want for no points! Maybe we should eat a lot more vegetables to lose weight and feel healthier.

Very Thin and Overweight are Protein Filled

Weight is an inaccurate measurement of being healthy. Even though an individual may have lost 100 pounds and may be healthier from a weight stand point, they are probably still severely acidic, full of protein and unknowingly unhealthy. We can be either very thin or overweight and still be acidic and protein filled. If you are thin the proteins may be congesting your blood vessels, bones or organs.

I have been on diets most of my life, always losing then gaining it back. In the past few years, for the first time in my life, I have been able to maintain less than 200 pounds (I was over 240) by eating more alkaline foods, doing some exercise and taking nutritional supplements. Daily self–lymphatic activation is a big key to losing weight and balancing your body. When I'm on vacation or have a few parties in a row I tend to eat more acid foods like meats, pasta, bread, beer or wine. I feel heavier immediately and begin to feel bloated, muscle tension, gas and itchy skin after a very acid or protein filled meal. To balance myself I then go on a 90% alkaline to 10% acid diet until I feel better. After a few times of seeing your problems go away with a better diet and then return with a more acidic diet, you smarten up and eat less acid and protein in your diet.

The New Government Food Pyramid

The Surgeon General feels Americans are overweight and is suggesting we eat smaller portions. Besides smaller portions, the government's food pyramid should have a little quotation on the pamphlet, "Remember the 80/20 Rule". The government food pyramid, which has served us for 15 years, has gone through a facelift. With the old pyramid we counted servings of the specific food groups. This has changed since the government feels the vagueness of the serving size has led to an overweight America.

In 2005 the pyramid took on a totally new design which I believe is confusing. It features rainbow-colored bands representing different food groups, running from the pyramid's top to the bottom instead of horizontally. We no longer count servings of the different food groups but count ounces or cups. Grains are still the largest portion, but they emphasize to eat half of your daily allotment of grains as whole grains. Even though I believe this is a giant step in the right direction, I believe that grains, even whole grains are acid forming and should be eaten sparingly. White flour products should be avoided most of the time.

If you understand how the government works, watching out for corporate interests, suggesting to eat some whole grain products, is probably done to appease the lobbyists and companies that produce processed white flour products. Your health is less important than corporate interests. Vegetables and then fruits are next on the pyramid and then milk and after that meat and beans. A better food pyramid begins with fruits and vegetables as its base, then healthy oils, alkaline nuts and limited whole grains, then beans, chicken, fish then beef and other processed acid forming foods should remain the smallest portion.

Now that you know about acid-alkaline foods you can see that the government is still recommending that we eat grains, an acid forming food, as our main staple. This misguided advice is helping fuel the nation's health crisis. If you want help with the new government food pyramid there is a 70 page booklet to help explain it to you. If it takes 70 pages to explain, it's too difficult to understand. Or you can just balance your intake to 80% alkaline foods to 20% acid foods.

An Out of Balanced Body Will Tolerate Acid and Other Toxins

In my opinion, the reason we don't realize that our acidic diet is hurting us is because our body has had to deal with excess acid and protein since we were very young, possibly within the womb. We are already congested and don't realize the additional congestion we feel from acidic foods until we become overly toxic or protein filled. Your body is very good at adapting to things that are not good for you. Look at how the body will tolerate cocaine, crack, meth, marijuana, alcohol, coffee, chocolate and processed white flour, these are all acid forming in the body. You will feel your worst fatigue, pain, anxiety or depression when you are severely overly acidic and toxic. I have seen this over and over again in our wellness center. The remainder of the time your body is dealing with moderate acidity with stomach problems, mild headaches, aches from arthritis, inability to sleep or recurring infections.

If you are severely acidic, green your diet and go through a few series of lymphatic activation sessions in order to rid your body of acid wastes. As your tissues become more balanced your body will not tolerate excess acid as easily. After you eat an acidic meal, you will begin to feel your shoulders, low back or buttock muscles tighten as the cellular environment becomes more acidic. Your cells don't like being in a toxic environment.

Processed Foods are Not Good for You

Eating processed foods such as white rice, white flour products or highly processed products with many food additives, will add to your toxicity. Eat foods in their natural form. Instead of using canned vegetables or fruits use fresh or frozen for your meals. Frozen foods are fully ripened and then quickly processed and flash frozen. In the processing of rice and wheat we remove the shell or germ, which is where most of the nutrition is. This wheat bran or germ is actually given to livestock for added nutrition or sold to us as wheat germ. Processed wheat flour is often bleached white to make it more appealing. Very often you will see the words "fortified" for white flour products. This is because processing removes the natural nutrition so they fortify the flour with cheap supplements. So look in your cabinets and start to become more aware of how often you are eating processed food or more nutritious food.

CHAPTER FIFTEEN

Tips on Eating "80/20"

A New Look at Food

We need to start looking at our food differently, it's not to just to fill us up, it's meant to give us nutrition, a power source. When we concentrate on eating till we become full we over eat. We should concentrate on eating less food but more nutritious food. This begins with breakfast; typically you are told that breakfast is the most important meal, so you load up. If you start your day with large amounts of acid foods like eggs, bacon, toast, oatmeal, bagels, coffee or orange juice you are over loading your system first thing in the morning. This adds to congestion in the body. Your day should start with a light nutritious meal of fresh fruits or fresh fruit and vegetable juice on most days. Try slices of apples or celery with almond butter for breakfast or a snack.

More Fruits and Vegetables

We have to be realistic; there may not be a perfect diet, food or snack. The goal is to eat more unprocessed foods and more nutritious foods (fruits, vegetables and some whole grains). In preparing your meals you may use a small amount of acid forming ingredients such as vinegar, black pepper, certain beans, meat, fish, chicken and even ketchup. Remember to keep acid forming foods to around 20% of your diet. As more of the public learns about acid-alkaline balance, producers of food products will have to produce more alkaline forming products, even snacks.

Buy a Vegetarian Cookbook

Since you will be eating more vegetables, buy a good vegetarian cookbook o start collecting vegetarian recipes from the Internet. Take some of your family recipes and make them healthier by removing some of the meat and adding more vegetables. Even vegetarian recipes will have to be changed a little to make them more alkaline like using brown rice or Quinoa instead of white rice.

Don't Leave the House Without a Nutritious Snack

Whenever you are out of the house, pack a small cooler with water, some fruit, raw vegetables or healthy snacks to take with you. It always happens, especially if you have kids. You are out shopping or running errands and they get hungry. The next thing you know you are pulling into a fast food drive-thru. Being prepared with healthy snacks will help keep you out of the drive-thru and keep you and your children healthier. At first the kids may grumble and want the drive thru if that is what they are used to having. Be consistent with having your own healthy food and snacks and the kids will get used to the new way of eating.

Eat Some Vegetables Raw

Eating some of your vegetables raw, or slightly steamed, is very healthy. Vegetables that have been cooked over 118 degrees Fahrenheit lose their enzymes. Enzymes are very important to your overall well being. They act as a catalyst for many of your metabolic functions. Cooking vegetables is not the only way to damage enzymes. When a vegetable is picked to go to market, it has 100% of its enzymatic potential. Within a few hours the enzymatic potential can be as low as 50%. Many of our fruits and vegetables sit in large warehouses for a week or more before they reach a supermarket, and as a result have little enzymatic potential. This is why you need to incorporate fresh raw vegetables and systemic enzymes into your diet.

In our refrigerator we try and keep some raw vegetables ready to eat for convenience. Some examples are a sweet and spicy Napa cabbage salad, roasted red peppers in olive oil and garlic, whole radishes, steamed broccoli, home made pickles in salt brine without vinegar, as well as gazpacho (a mix-re of fresh tomatoes, green pepper, cucumber, onion, cilantro, avocado, olive lime juice and sea salt). Gazpacho is a great, fresh tasting, cold chunky I love to eat a cup of gazpacho before my meals or as a snack. It's full of ns and minerals. Try to only use fresh ingredients in your gazpacho, no omato juice.

Eat a Salad Shortly Before Your Meal or as a Meal

Many people have problems digesting lettuce and there is a reason for this. Lettuce is full of water and alkalizing. When you eat salad with a meal or right after, it dilutes the acid in your stomach and slows your digestion. You should eat a salad before the main meal, on an empty stomach, so it will move through the system faster and not interfere with the digestion of your meal. Salads can be more than a starter, add a few vegetables and you have a healthy meal.

Eat Fruit on an Empty Stomach

Fruits digest very quickly. If we eat them right after a meal they start to break down, resting on top of the heavier food that takes longer to digest. The fruit can ferment and create more acid waste and gas. Fasting on fruit is detoxifying.

Have More Fruits and Vegetables Cut Up and Ready To Eat

I find it amazing that a whole melon will sit on the counter for days. When it's cut up and put it into the refrigerator we all begin to pick at it. It has to be convenient.

Eat Brown Rice Instead of White

White rice has been processed and has little nutritional value compared to brown rice, which has sometimes double or triple the alkaline forming minerals of white rice. Brown rice comes to us with the hull and germ. This hull and germ are full of vitamins and minerals. White rice has been processed to remove the hull and germ, which removes much of the nutritional value. Aid organizations can use this knowledge to truly benefit millions. We send processed white rice to starving nations or for disaster relief. White rice is very acid forming and causes bloating. A simple change of sending brown rice we would be doubling or tripling the nutrition given to these people who are suffering from malnutrition.

You may think that changing from white rice to brown rice is a simple matter. For most of you it will be an easy switch, once you know that brown rice is much healthier than white rice. America is a melting pot of many different cultures. Some cultural beliefs have strong ties that go back thousands of years. In many areas around the world, specifically Asia and The Middle East, white rice is part of their culture. It is time to look at new information that will improve the health of your future generations.

Grow Your Own Sprouts

People have been growing sprouts for thousands of years. Instead of planting a seed and letting it grow to maturity, the seed is soaked and allowed to sprout, turning green in a few days. They are full of vitamins, minerals and enzymes. It takes only a few days to grow sprouts in a jar in your kitchen. Some common varieties are alfalfa, chickpea, broccoli, almond, green lentil and buckwheat. You can eat them on sandwiches, in salads or alone as a nutritious snack. Most health food stores have sprouting kits and supplies.

Sprouted or Whole Wheat Breads and Tortillas

As a nation we eat a large amount of bread, especially our children. By eating whole-wheat products you are consuming a more nutritious product, but not necessarily alkalizing. Since the Government food pyramid now suggests we eat more whole grains, more companies are making healthier whole grain products. Be sure to read the labels. Many products that claim to be whole-wheat may contain processed bleached white flour as the main ingredient. Many of the soft whole-wheat breads found in supermarkets contain many other ingredients such as dough conditioners and preservatives. More traditional breads are made of whole grains, water, yeast and salt. Sprouted breads are made from young sprouted seeds that are alive and full of nutrition. These healthier breads tend to be hardier than the soft white bread we are accustomed to. There are many types of sprouted or whole-wheat breads to choose from, try a few in order to find one you like. Overall eat less grains.

Quinoa – A Super Food

Try eating more quinoa (pronounced KEEN-WAH), it is a good source of easily digestible protein. Quinoa is not a grain but a seed from a plant similar to spinach. It has a nutty flavor that is prepared and eaten like rice. Unlike rice or grains, quinoa has a balanced set of amino acids and contains no gluten. Its texture is softer more delicate than rice, when you chew it you feel a little pop in your mouth almost like al dente pasta.

Healthier Pasta

We eat a great deal of pasta in our society, it is acid forming in your body. I previously ate pasta three or four times a week. Now that I know it increases my acidity I eat it less often. Thankfully, large companies are beginning to understand acid-alkaline balance. Pasta companies are now making multigrain pasta with semolina or whole-wheat flour.

One company that is leading the way is Barilla. This company has made their Barilla Plus line of pasta more nutritious than traditional pasta. Their pasta is made from Durum Wheat, oats, spelt, barley, lentils, chickpeas and flax seeds. Compared to traditional pasta, in my opinion Barilla Plus is a super food, because they made the pasta more nutritious. It tastes like regular pasta; you just need to soften the pasta by cooking it a little longer after it is done.

Fresher Pasta Sauces

White flour pasta is acid forming and if we eat it with canned tomato sauce we are now eating two acidic foods. Making a tomato sauce from fresh tomatoes, not canned, is healthier for you. You can add a pinch or two of baking soda to your tomato sauce to cut the acidity, too much will ruin your sauce. Try greening up your sauces. A great basic sauce is aglio e olio (garlic and oil). Sauté olive oil, garlic, a little crushed red pepper and course sea salt until the garlic is slightly golden. Slightly steam some mixed vegetables, place into the olive oil and garlic mixture and saute for a minute or two, place on top of cooked pasta. Add a big handful of chopped basil to make it even healthier.

Green Up Eggs

Instead of eating eggs alone, add potato, onions, peppers, spinach or broccoli, which are all alkaline. Eggs are an easily digestible protein source; a large egg provides 6 grams of protein. Eggs have the highest quality protein in the food supply with the amino acid pattern almost matching the human requirement for essential amino acids.

Cut Down On Bread

Wrap tuna salad, deli meats or grilled vegetables in a piece of lettuce instead of using bread or a tortilla. In & Out Burger serves a protein burger that is not on the menu. The burger is made the same way, but instead of a bun they wrap it with lettuce leaves. When eating fast food remove the bread from one side of the sandwich to cut down on the bread.

Greener Sandwiches

When making a sandwich use whole-grain or sprouted bread. Cut down on the amount of meat and cheese and add extra tomatoes, avocado, roasted red peppers, onion, green peppers, jalapenos, cabbage or lettuce.

When Having Oatmeal, Add Raisins

Oatmeal is acid forming. When using the 5-minute oatmeal instead of the instant, throw a big handful of raisins into your water while cooking. They make a nice alkaline addition to your breakfast. Try not to eat oatmeal everyday.

Lemon Juice and Water Between Meals

For decades many health books have recommended that you drink lemon juice in water. Lemons are very acidic but in the body they have an alkalizing affect. There is no clear explanation for why this occurs. One reason may be that lemons have a large amount of minerals, which makes them more alkalizing. It may be that the acidity of the lemon is like Drain-O and opens our circulation. If you get back pain, drink a large glass or two of water with the juice of half a lemon over a few minutes. Your pain will diminish and within a half hour you will feel the need to urinate. You may notice your urine stream will be heavier than usual. Remember balance is the key.

Eat Potatoes

You have been told that potatoes, a carbohydrate, are bad for you so many barely eat them. A medium potato supplies 610 mg. of potassium and other nutrients, 3-9 grams of protein and 2.3 grams of fiber. For digestive problems, potatoes, especially when eaten slightly raw in the center or juiced raw, have strong healing powers. Now my family will eat at least five pounds of potatoes a week. For breakfast we may have sautéed potatoes with green pepper and onion or potato pancakes. Lunch could be a salad of steamed fresh green beans and potato with garlic and olive oil. For dinner we may have a large salad with potato soup. We do have the occasional meat and potatoes. Sweet potatoes and yams are more nutritious than white potatoes.

Avocados, Radishes, Mangos, Kiwi's and Figs are Very Alkalinizing

I was amazed to see how nutritious many of the above fruits are, especially avocados. We very rarely ate them until I learned that they are so healthy. Avocados contain three to four times the nutrition of other fruits and vegetables. They provide an impressive 1204 mg. of potassium, bananas supply 467 mg. and apples supply 158 mg. of potassium. Although the banana is thought of as a good source of potassium you can see the avocado actually supplies much more. Avocados contain a healthy fat that is highly monounsaturated, the kind that's associated with a healthy heart. They are high in fiber, protein and provide substantial amounts of magnesium, folate (folic acid), vitamin B6, and pantothenic acid, as well as some iron and copper. Avocados also contain glutathione, an antioxidant with anti-carcinogenic powers.

Eat Almonds

Many of the nuts we eat, like cashews and peanuts, are acid forming. Instead of giving up on nuts entirely, try eating almonds or Brazil nuts. They are more alkaline and are full of protein, magnesium, vitamin E, riboflavin and healthy monounsaturated fats. Store almonds in the refrigerator in a container, when you are ready to have a handful, toss some in the toaster oven for 30 seconds.

Alkaline Snacks

Besides fruits and vegetables, many stores carry healthier crackers made with whole-wheat, brown rice, quinoa or almonds. Because you are eating more fruits and vegetables, you crave something that crunches in your mouth. Jicama, celery or cucumbers can be sliced and added to salads or eaten alone, with guacamole or almond butter. Some of my favorite snacks are melons, dried figs and dried peas with wasabi. As more companies learn about acid-alkaline balance you will see a larger variety of alkalizing snacks and other products available in more than just health food stores.

Juicing

Fresh vegetable and fruit juices are full of vitamins and minerals and are very alkalizing to your body. Fresh squeezed orange, grapefruit and tomato juice are alkaline, but when they are processed they become acid forming. In the morning I enjoy fresh juice from a combination of fresh fruits and vegetables. My favorite juice is made from apples, carrots, celery and beets. If you don't have the time to juice them yourself, there are many companies that are producing fruit and vegetable drinks from puree that they call super foods. Odwalla is one company that is in most supermarkets. Avoid or limit juices that are too sweet or are made from concentrate.

Fruit Smoothies

Fruit smoothies are a great way to get kids and adults to have fruit and water at the same time. In a blender place a peeled banana, half of a cup of natural apple juice, a combination of frozen fruits and ice, blend together for a great tasting, hydrating, healthy snack.

Vegetable Broth

Homemade vegetable broth is very alkalizing to your body and is full of vitamins and minerals. As you begin to eat more vegetables, you may have more unused raw vegetables in the refrigerator. Instead of throwing them out, make a vegetable broth and freeze it into small containers for later use. The nutritious broth can be added to many foods such as in mashed potatoes, soups, stews or used in pasta sauces. It's also great as a hot beverage all by itself. If you don't have the time to make your own vegetable broth, purchase one that has only limited ingredients like filtered water, vegetables and sea salt.

Herbal Teas

We are accustomed to drinking black, Oolong and Earl Grey teas. Green teas are popular and are hyped for their antioxidants. Most of these teas are acid forming, especially drinks with green tea and high fructose corn syrup. A better choice would be herbal teas. Many of the teas that say herbal are traditional brown or green teas with herbs. This is not what you want. True herbal teas are made from alkalizing herbs such as chicory, rose hips, hibiscus flowers, lemon peel and fruit. Try making your own healthy tea made from a few sprigs of fresh parsley, a few bay leaves or mint in hot water.

Herbal Coffee

In Caffeine Blues, by nutritional biochemist Stephen Cherniske, he explains how caffeine can aggravate heart disease, diabetes, acid indigestion, insomnia, PMS, depression, anxiety, stress, fatigue, blood sugar swings and many other health problems. Coffee is very acid forming in your body. Many need a daily fix of two or three cups of coffee. This is very acid forming and unhealthy and can lead to impeded circulation and fatigue in the body.

Herbal coffee is a blend of alkaline herbs, nuts, fruits and grains that are roasted, ground and brewed just like coffee. One company that I like is Teeccino. Their healthy blends contain 65mg of potassium to give you a natural lift and 365mg of inulin, a soluble fiber in chicory root, that helps improve digestion and elimination plus increases the absorption of calcium and minerals. My wife needed her coffee to get through the day. She was able to make a smooth transition from coffee to herbal coffee and does not miss the regular coffee. Recently she had a cup of regular coffee and didn't like how it made her feel. She felt jittery and ill. Keep trying different herbal coffees until you find one that you like.

There are some individuals who can drink coffee or espresso before bed. Their body is so accustomed to the acidity and caffeine that they don't feel the negative affects of the coffee. Even though you may not feel the negative affects, such as limiting your circulation or constricting your tissues, it is still happening. Try not drinking coffee for a month and then see how your cleaner body reacts to the acidic coffee and caffeine. Drinking decaffeinated coffee is not much better for you than regular coffee. It is still an acidic beverage. It may actually be worse for you due to the solvents left in the bean after the decaffeinating process.

Sea Salt

Salt is an essential component to good health. Processed salt will limit your health. The processing of salt strips it of many of its beneficial elements like minerals. Sea salt is a better more complete and healthier choice that does not contribute to high blood pressure.

Heavy Protein Meal Take Enzymes

When you know you are going to eat a high animal protein meal take a few digestive or systemic enzymes to help digest the heavy protein. This is really an important step in reducing cellular waste from accumulating in your body.

Some Basic Dietary Help

I really feel it is the science of how acid is slowing the lymphatic system allowing proteins (cell material) to fill the body that is important to understand. By being too acidic you are actually filling with your own cellular waste. You have the choice to follow the following routine as strictly or as loosely as you want for 15 to 30 days. This only details the dietary component of the 5 Steps, be sure to include increasing your circulation, good posture, deep breathing, enough good water, stress reduction and lymphatic activation.

Week One

Buy a good vegetarian cookbook or go to the Internet for vegetarian recipes. Your goal in the first week is to become familiar with eating close to 80% alkaline (fruits and vegetables) and 20% acid foods and drink (allows for some acid foods). Eat six smaller meals throughout the day and begin to eat less processed foods, sodas, coffee and tea. Don't worry if you fall off the wagon the first week, you are anxious about not being able to eat the foods you love, just get up and start again. Once you have detoxed and balanced your body you will be eating your normal foods (even fast food) just not as often. First we need to detox the body by eating almost all alkaline foods to eliminate years of trapped waste and replenish minerals into the body.

Week Two

Go to a 90% alkaline and 10% acid food diet, a little fish and chicken, no wheat or grains. Stop processed foods, sodas, coffee, tea and alcohol.

Week Three

Eliminate meat, chicken and fish, just fruits, vegetables and alkaline nuts. This may sound difficult but with some meal planning it can become a welcome break from years of eating excess meat protein. The key is to stay focused on the end result a cleaner, healthier body.

Week Four

A fast of vegetable broth and a lemonade fast (a combination of maple syrup, lemon juice and cayenne pepper) lasting between 3-7 days. Even though you will lose weight the fast is for detoxing the body not for weight loss. Once drinking liquids during the fast you will not look for food. Come out of the fast slowly and try and maintain close to an "80/20 Diet." More details on fasting in the next chapter.

CHAPTER SIXTEEN

Diet Alone is Not Enough!

When Not to Eat and Much Needed Nutritional Support

Fasting: A Fresh Start

We have talked about what foods to eat. Now let's discuss when there is a time not to eat. The idea of not eating, or fasting, has been used to increase health for thousands of years. Fasting helps to clean your blood, tissues and organs of acidic wastes and proteins that have congested your body and slowed your circulation. I believe fasting for 7 to 10 days or more, every two months, is an easy way to help keep your body from becoming congested. Even though you haven't eaten any solid foods during the fast, your body will continue to assimilate whatever remains within it. Without the burden of solid foods, your body systems can digest and clean deeper than when working to digest your daily consumption of highly acid forming and high protein foods and drinks.

The breakdown of stored or circulating waste and proteins is the basic process of detoxification. During a fast, the tissues, blood and lymph have the opportunity to be cleaned of waste and toxins. The interstitial fluid becomes cleaner and each cell has the opportunity to clean its toxic, acidic waste and take in oxygen and nutrition to repair itself.

On the 10th day of my last fast from food, I had gone to have some blood drawn for testing. The lab technician and I couldn't believe my blood was so watery. Normally it flows out like syrup, but this time it shot to the back of the vial. During a fast your body continues to clean the waste and excess proteins from your blood, tissues and organs.

There are many different types of fasts. One that I have used often is "The Master Cleanser" by Stanley Burroughs. This basic seven-day fast begins with the consumption of fruits and raw vegetables on day one, fresh fruit juices on day two (avoid juices from concentrate and acidic juices such as processed orange or grapefruit juices). Days three, four and five, or longer, you can have homemade vegetable broth and a lemonade mixture throughout the day. Have at least eight glasses of the lemonade mixture per day.

This healthy lemonade will be giving you the majority of your vitamins and minerals for the day. It is prepared using 8 ounces of water, two tablespoons of fresh lemon juice (or the juice of half a lemon), 2 tablespoons of dark amber maple syrup and one tenth of a teaspoon of ground cayenne pepper (the mixture tastes similar to lemonade with a kick). On day six you start back with fruit juices, day seven you eat fruits and then raw vegetables. Start day eight with some fruits then vegetables and you will be ready for some light food by evening. If the mixture is too sweet use only 1 tblsp. of maple syrup.

Fasting Tips

Adding essential fatty acids (EFA's) to your fast is a good idea because they are important for proper brain and nerve function. When I am fasting, I take a tablespoon of olive oil, coconut oil or a few capsules of fish oil daily. During the fast you will feel healthier and have less of your symptoms. While on the fast avoid strenuous or prolonged exercise. Since you haven't eaten you don't have the large amounts of nutrients necessary to fuel your body during heavy or prolonged exertion. There are many ways to fast and it is advisable to buy a book on the subject or research it on the Internet. Remember, during a fast the body still needs nutrition. A fast with just water is too drastic and can hurt your cells. A modified fast can consist of eating fruits and raw vegetables or fresh fruit juice and fresh vegetable juices for a few days to a week.

Most people worry that they will be hungry during a fast. Once you stop eating and are taking in only liquids, you will no longer look for food if you are drinking enough lemonade mixture. Even though you will lose weight the goal in fasting is to clean your body, increase your health and lower your risk of disease. Drinking water throughout the day is very important during a fast. Your body and organs function best when they are fully hydrated. Never break a fast and start eating solid foods. You will have severe abdominal cramping and be running to the restroom for days. Always ease your way back to solid foods over a few days.

If you are very sick, consult your doctor so you can work together to monitor you during the fast. Pregnant or nursing mothers should not fast but should definitely slowly change their diet by increasing their intake to more fruits, vegetables and water.

Diet Alone is Not a Cure

Even though eating a greener diet is an important part of good health, most vegetarians, or people who say they have changed their diet to include healthier foods, are shocked when they test severely acidic. For this exact reason I believe strongly that diet changes alone will have only a limited effect on your pH and overall health. It takes many changes in lifestyle choices in addition to a greener diet, like nutritional supplements (especially alkalizing and proteolytic products), daily exercise, increased hydration, deep breathing, stress reduction and lymphatic activation to help bring you back to balance. When you take alkalizing supplements and systemic enzymes, you may feel a slight acid feeling in your stomach after a half-hour of taking the supplements. This is the body beginning to move acid waste out of the tissues. Drink some water to flush the body and the feeling goes away.

Basic Nutritional Supplementation

Multivitamin

Your health is dependent on vitamins, and especially minerals, circulating through your tissues. The body is like a high performance engine that needs high octane, fuel to run properly. Natural and whole foods such as fruits, vegetables and herbs that contain vitamins, minerals and micro-nutrients are good fuel. Avoid synthetic vitamins that don't have the micro-nutrients that help vitamins and minerals work. Very often I hear people say that they are taking vitamins A, C and E. If you don't have the minerals and micro-nutrients many of your vitamins won't absorb or work efficiently. We should all be taking some type of multivitamin and mineral supplement. It's an insurance policy that helps to fill in the voids within your diet. Balance is more important than potency.

A 1999 Harvard Report on Cancer Prevention showed that men and women who took a multivitamin containing folic acid cut their risk of colon cancer by 50%. In a Nurses' Health Study, women who took multivitamins for at least 15 years were 75% less likely to develop colon cancer than women who never took multivitamins.

It amazes me that with all this positive information about multivitamin use, I often hear people say they have been told that "vitamins are a waste of money." The studies show a multivitamin alone can cut your risk of disease. What will happen if you start eating more fruits and vegetables and begin taking more alkalizing products that contain large amounts of vitamins and minerals? I believe this will slowly build your mineral reserve and ultimately make you more alkaline and healthier.

More than One a Day

There are many multivitamins on the market to choose from. You don't need to spend a fortune to get good protection. You do have to realize that if you look for a bargain price multivitamin you may not be getting everything that you need. Look for companies that are keeping up with technology by adding more magnesium or a less acidic form of Vitamin C called Ester-C. Multivitamins that only provide the RDA (Required Daily Allowance) are giving you minimal amounts of nutrients, just enough to keep you from becoming sick but not actually enough to make you healthy.

Look for a multivitamin that provides the Suggested Optimal Daily Nutritional Allowances (SONA), which is often much more than the RDA. You need more than a one a day multivitamin. Your body needs nutrition throughout the day, even while you are sleeping. Find a multivitamin where you take one or two capsules in the morning as well as in the evening to insure that proper nutrition is available to your body as it needs it.

I feel comfortable recommending Perfect Multi Super Greens by Purity Products. It delivers the antioxidant equivalent of 7-9 servings of fruits and vegetables per serving. Super Greens is an optimally balanced blend of dark greens, phytonutrients, as well as vitamins and minerals.

Stress Formula

If you feel you are under a great deal of stress (who isn't these days), look for a multivitamin formula designed for stress or add a stress formula to your vitamin and mineral regime. Most stress formulations will have extra B vitamins, extra vitamin C and minerals such as magnesium or zinc. I especially like combinations that also contain herbs that are known to relax us, like passion flower or valerian root.

Magnesium

Magnesium is one of the most overlooked minerals in your body. It is perhaps the most vital mineral. When there is a deficiency of magnesium, the body will not function properly. The National Institute of Health describes magnesium as a mineral needed by every cell. It is necessary for more than 300 biochemical reactions in the body. It helps maintain normal muscle and nerve function, keeps your heart rhythm steady and helps to keep your bones strong. It is also very important for energy metabolism and protein synthesis.

Not only is it critical for energy production and proper nerve function, it also helps to relax your muscles and assist the body in the production and use of insulin. The American Diabetes Association announced that a diet rich in magnesium might help prevent Type 2 Diabetes. Magnesium helps to alkalize your tissues to create a healthier cellular environment. Magnesium is often used to treat such ailments as back pain, high blood pressure, depression, anxiety, muscle cramps, arrhythmias, constipation and migraines. Magnesium is nature's own calcium channel blocker. When there is enough magnesium present, your arteries and veins relax or dilate. This lessens resistance and improves the flow of lymph and blood. This increases the body's ability to cleanse itself and to deliver oxygen and nutrients throughout the body.

Magnesium Relaxes You

My first experience with magnesium was during a very stressful time in my life. My heart would race and felt as though it would beat right out of my chest. After a few weeks of this I saw an ad for Natural Calm by Peter Gillham's Natural Vitality. It is a highly absorbable form of magnesium citrate. The ad mentioned that many of our common health problems are caused by magnesium deficiency. It even mentioned palpitations. I ordered the product and when it arrived I put a heaping teaspoon in 4 ounces of hot water. The mixture began to fizz. I let it cool a little and proceeded to drink the warm mineral tasting water. Later that same night the pounding in my chest was gone.

When I forget to take magnesium for a few days, my feet begin to become tight and sore. The muscles in my shoulders and low back also begin to tighten. When I begin to feel tightness in my body, I have come to the realization that I am receiving a warning that I am becoming too acidic and toxic. Natural Calm is one of my favorite products. People who have pain, heart problems, insomnia, migraines, depression, anxiety or low energy need magnesium. Recently, a customer came into our wellness center and noticed the Natural Calm for sale. She said she had just switched heart doctors and her new doctor, who is more holistic, took her off a few medications and gave her Natural Calm. She has been able to control her heart problem with magnesium and much less medication. When taking extra magnesium make sure your diet and multivitamin includes calcium to balance the magnesium. I especially like a product called Natural Calm with Calcium also by Peter Gillham's Natural Vitality. A synergistic blend of magnesium, calcium, potassium, Vitamin C, Vitamin D3 and boron. A more balanced product.

Buffer Your Acid

Buffer pH+, created by Vaxa International, is a homeopathic formulation that assists the body naturally and safely in balancing an overly acid system. The alkalizing complexes and phytonutrients within Buffer pH+ help buffer and remove overly acidic wastes from the body. Millions of us are out of balance and have acid related health problems. I believe this product should be a part of everybody's alkalizing regime. Information on the bottle indicates that it also "Aids in Weight Loss." When you are more alkaline, your lymphatic system can remove excess fluid and waste that forms fat in the body. Buffer pH+ was one of the first alkalizing products I started to utilize and within a few weeks I started to feel a difference. By using Vaxa's Buffer pH+, as well as exercising and maintaining a greener diet, I began losing weight and experiencing less stomach problems, especially bloating and irritable bowel syndrome (IBS).

Balance Not Potency

SeaAloe is a balanced whole food nutritional supplement with plant based ingredients that is in an easily assimilated cherry tasting liquid. Its proprietary blend of aloe vera, Pau D'Arco Extract, blend of seven sea vegetables and four concentrated juices (cranberry, concord grape, white grape and black cherry are a powerful alkalizer and delivers over 80 vitamins, minerals, trace minerals and amino acids in Nature's Perfect Balance.

This product is perfect for those that don't want to bother with a lot of products. I especially like this product because it is a very safe product for those on medications, pregnant and children. Always check with your physician if you have any health conditions. I saw my child's constipation and eczema leave after only a few weeks of using SeaAloe. Remember too much of even a good thing could be hazardous to your health. Even though this is a very gentle product, it is powerful. Start with small doses of SeaAloe, half an ounce twice a day for a few days, then an ounce twice a day. Drink water after you take it to assist in the cleansing that will take place. My children who are five and six take half the recommended dosage twice per day. SeaAloe contains whole food natural ingredients that are helpful in gently alkalizing, remineralizing and cleansing the cells and tissues of the body. When your body is more alkaline the cells which make up everything in your body, have a healthier environment. This can positively influence your overall health. My children were on a very similar product for three weeks before I switched to SeaAloe. The first night after taking 1/2 ounce of SeaAloe my daughter broke out in an itchy rash on her chest and back. To most people this may have been alarming but I understood that her body was cleaning itself. This reaction in my daughter showed me how powerful SeaAloe is. When we become more alkaline, trapped toxins are being released from the tissues. After the third night of SeaAloe her rash went away.

Essential Fatty Acids

Essential Fatty Acids (EFA's) are necessary fats that humans cannot manufacture and must be obtained through diet. There are two families of EFA's we need to consume: Omega-3 and Omega-6. Your diet now includes huge amounts of Omega-6 oils that are extracted from plants and used for cooking or in prepared foods. These oils (such as corn oil, safflower oil, cottonseed oil, peanut oil, soybean oil) are primarily Omega-6's. We have decreased our intake of Omega-3's, which are found primarily in whole grains, seafood, beans and other seeds. We should include more Omega 3's in our diet. EFA's are necessary for the formation of healthy cell membranes, the proper development and functioning of the brain and nervous system, as well as for the production of hormone-like substances. These chemicals regulate numerous body functions including blood pressure, blood viscosity and vasoconstriction, as well as immune and inflammatory responses. Ingesting too much Omega-6 and too little Omega-3 causes clots and constricts arteries, which increases the risk of heart attacks, increases edema and symptoms of arthritis as well as aggravates the skin disease psoriasis.

The best way to get your essential oils is through diet by eating more almonds, avocados, wild salmon, tuna and sardines. To fill in the gaps within your diet, you can take fish oil capsules or an EFA combination that may have flax oil, borage oil, coconut oil, and fish oils, these are all alkalizing to the body. It is very important for pregnant and nursing mothers to supplement their diets with EFA's. They are important to help maintain healthy developing cells, especially in the brain and nervous system. If you are feeding your infant by bottle you can place one or two drops of flax seed or fish oil in the formula. Look for fish oils that have gone through a molecular distillation process to remove toxins.

Green Products

When you go to your neighborhood health food store or shop online, you will be amazed at how many products are available to help you become more alkaline. They can range from a single herb like alfalfa to combinations of green vegetables, alkaline grasses or herbs. Green products are very alkalizing due to their high mineral content. It is very important to have many alkalizing products in your house to help balance your tissues. Here are a few ideas:

Liquid Chlorophyll - Chlorophyll is the ingredient in plants that make them green and is responsible for photosynthesis (converting light to energy). Consuming chlorophyll in a liquid form is a convenient and inexpensive way to get small amounts of easily digestible vitamins and minerals. Most liquid chlorophyll drinks are mint flavored and are made from alfalfa. Because of their long roots, alfalfa has a high mineral content and is used in many herbal combinations.

Super Green Products - These are products that are highly alkalizing and are concentrated forms of green foods such as broccoli, asparagus, alfalfa, Jerusalem artichoke, spirulina, wheat grass, barley grass, or any combination of fruits, vegetables and herbs. They come in capsule or powdered form that you can mix with water or organic natural fruit juice. These green powders are super foods that are an easy way to consume large amounts of naturally occurring enzymes, vitamins and minerals.

One product that I like is Greens Today. It is formulated and distributed by The Organic Frog, Inc. This company has a product line that is the only advanced 72 ingredient phytonutrient rich superfood designed to provide optimally balanced nutritional support from enzymatically active and alive foods. I like their vegan formula because it is the most alkalizing of their products and it supplies 1800 mg. of certified organic spirulina and 2000 mg. broccoli powder per serving. I like it shaken with water and a little organic apple juice. Your body needs alkalizing superfoods like this floating through your blood stream and into your tissues and organs to buffer acid waste and help you heal.

Another green drink that I like because of its good taste and amount of nutrition is Triple Greens by Purity Products. This all natural fruit and vegetable blend provides a full array of phytonutrients that powerfully support energy levels, heart health, brain health and a healthy immune system. Each scoop of Triple Greens contains 5000+ ORAC units (the antioxidant equivalent of 9+ servings of fruits and vegetables). Instead of substituting a heavy protein drink for a meal, substitute with a green drink, that is full of nutrition not proteins. There are some people who will not drink a green tasting drink. Purity Products has an answer, Perfect Purples. It's a delicious phytonutrient drink that combines 19 powerful exotic fruits and vegetables including Acai, Gogi and Mangosteen. It tastes great.

Systemic Enzymes

Enzymes are proteins that make life possible. They are necessary for thousands of chemical reactions to occur within your body. Without enzymes, little activity at all would take place. Vitamins, minerals and hormones won't work effectively without enzymes. They are present in all living cells where they perform a vital function by controlling the metabolic processes where nutrients are converted into energy and fresh cell material. Enzymes also take part in the breakdown of food materials into simpler compounds. Enzymes are biocatalysts, this means that by their mere presence, enzymes can speed up chemical processes that would otherwise happen very slowly in the body. Unfortunately enzyme production in the body begins to slow at age 27. This is when many of our aches and pains begin.

One of the most important roles of systemic enzymes is their proteolytic properties. Meaning they lyse or eat proteins like scar tissue or fibrosis in the body. An acidic pH and malfunctioning lymphatic system are creating protein proliferation in the body. Systemic enzymes are an important part to removing trapped proteins and opening your circulation. Basic digestive enzymes are specific, to be taken with a meal to help breakdown food in your system.

Systemic enzymes are more powerful than digestive enzymes. When taken on an empty stomach these enzymes go through the body lysing or eating excess proteins in your system that are congesting your circulation and may be causing pain or inflammation. Many of today's prescribed or over the counter anti-inflammatory medications may be dangerous to your health. Some have already been removed from the market. Enzymes are anti-inflammatory, and reduce pain and swelling.

When you start looking for systemic enzyme blends you need to know that there are basically two types, vegetarian and non-vegetarian. The vegetarian blends include papain, bromelain, protease, amylase, lipase and serrapeptidase. The enzymes in vegetarian formulations will be active in the body for 4-6 hours, so they should be taken three times a day. If you are not a vegetarian then you can take a non-vegetarian enzyme blend that contains the same enzymes papain, bromelain, protease, amylase, lipase and serrapeptase plus Trypsin and Chymotrypsin extracts from animal pancreatin. A benefit of using animal based pancreatin is its affordability and it's extended active life.

Research and clinical experience show that these enzyme blends last 24 to 36 hours in the body. That means most individuals taking a non-vegetarian blend of enzyme will be spending less and taking less pills than a vegetarian blend.

A non-vegetarian systemic enzyme blend that I highly recommend is Zymessence from WAM Essentials, Inc. For years I have taken 6-9 pills of a vegetarian enzyme blend and was satisfied with the results. What I especially like about Zymessence is its strength, affordability and the fact that I only take 2-4 pills a day.

Leaky Valves

A few years ago I injured my ankle for the fourth or fifth time in my life. After a few months, the leg started to feel tight and swollen. I went to my doctor and I was sent for a sonogram. I was diagnosed with leaky valves in my veins that were making my leg swell. For a year I wore a pressure stocking to keep the swelling down. When you injure yourself, the body sends out fibrin which over floods the area. This fibrin is similar to pieces of yarn that mix with cholesterol and cellular waste to clog your valves, vessels and tissues. After taking systemic enzymes for a few days my leg felt normal. As long as I take them I no longer have to wear a pressure stocking. If you have swelling, pain, inflammation or recurring infections you need to hydrate and take systemic enzymes to help increase your circulation.

Precaution: If you have a problem with blood clotting or are on a blood thinner, do not take systemic enzymes. Stop enzymes two weeks before any surgery.

CHAPTER SEVENTEEN

Step Three: Increase Your Circulation – Exercise, Deep Breathe, Hydrate And Posture

Circulation is the Answer

When it comes to your health it's really all about the circulation of oxygen, nutrients, and the removal of acid waste and excess proteins from around and in your cells. The "Big Question" is: In an overly acidic environment, are the cells able to receive oxygen and nutrition, and do they have the ability to move waste out of their cellular environment? Overly acidic tissues can become constricted, protein-filled and impede circulation. The reason you need to exercise is to increase circulation around and in your cells. Remember 500 million cells die daily, that adds up to a lot of waste in the body. When you increase circulation around your cells and through your tissues and organs, you increase the ability of the body to cleanse itself and heal.

Exercise contracts your muscles and makes you deep breathe. These actions also help to move lymph and blood through your tissues. Exercise increases circulation which forces oxygenated blood deeper into the microcirculation of the tissues. If you are sedentary, you are not pumping your heart strongly enough to move waste out of the tissues or organs. This increase in heart action is necessary to move the fluids in your tissues with enough force to move through the possibly millions of miles of blood and lymph vessels that are meant to support your cells and tissues. Without healthy circulation your cells and tissues become toxic and your health is negatively affected.

If You Don't Move You Lose

You need to exercise almost daily to efficiently move and detox your blood and body. In 1996 the U.S. Department of Health and Human Services issued the first-ever Surgeon General's Report on Physical Activity and Health. They recommended 30 minutes of moderate physical activity per day. The report found regular, moderate physical activity could substantially reduce the risk of premature death, heart disease, diabetes, colon cancer and high blood pressure as well as enhancing mental health. The report indicated that 60% of Americans are not regularly active. When you are sedentary, waste can build in your tissues and you can become overly acidic. Your tissues and vessels constrict causing your body to fill with waste and fluid. In evidence I point to the many diseases associated with excess fluid, swelling (edema), enlarged organs and fluid filled cysts that were mentioned in chapter one.

I recently had a ganglion cyst that would appear and disappear since I was a kid, removed from my right wrist. Within days another cyst had started to grow next to where the old one was. When an area is acidic or congested from protein, the 2–10% of fluid that is not being picked up by the slowed or stopped lymphatic system invades the tissue or organ. They removed my ganglion cyst but the fluid that was filling it was still present and began to fill the area and created another ganglion cyst. This excess fluid can invade your ovaries, prostate, lungs, brain and nerves. By repeatedly activating the lymphatics in my axilla and arm the ganglion cyst went away. If you have a tight pelvis or back you can be impeding the circulation of the nerves in your legs. The nerves can become acidic, protein filled and toxic, you may feel numbness and tingling, or it can feel as if it's on fire. Numbness and tingling is a sign of Amyloidosis, a buildup of abnormal proteins in the body.

There is an easy solution for most people with tingling sensations, loss of sensation or pain, simply increase the circulation in the problem area. If it hurts too much to exercise, start with a few light Swedish massages, CranioSacral Therapy or Lymph Drainage Therapy sessions. As you begin to feel better, find some exercises you can do that will increase overall body circulation, especially in your problem area. You are responsible for moving your blood to help clean your body.

What stops most people from continuing with a new exercise regime is an increase in their pain or fatigue. Patients tell me they stop exercising because of soreness or because they felt tired the next day. When you exercise, you are releasing toxins, waste and proteins that overwhelm your system (remember the healing crisis). To alleviate a healing crisis try an Epsom salt bath and keep exercising at a lower intensity while you are not feeling well. This can help to clear the excess toxins that were produced when you initially started exercising. You will feel better if you give it a chance.

Small Blockages Become Life Threatening Blockages

Many people are out walking, biking and going to the gym trying to keep healthy. They are trying to increase their circulation and trying to lower their risk of disease. Over acidity can impede your circulation by constricting the lymph vessels and creating excess proteins and waste in your tissues. These constricted vessels in your tissues may be as small as a strand of hair. They can become clogged with protein, cholesterol and waste creating soft blockages. The more you move, bend or deep breathe the more you are opening these soft blockages allowing circulation through the tissues and organs.

The problem occurs when you become less active, eat a highly acidic diet and become dehydrated. If you lead a sedentary lifestyle you may not be moving enough to keep these soft protein jams, made of dead cells, fibrin, minerals and cholesterol broken up. As this waste builds and becomes harder, it may form a blood clot and become life threatening. Being dehydrated creates more circulation problems due to less fluid volume in the body necessary for circulation. I like to equate our heart and many miles of vessels to a hydraulic pump and a plumbing system. If you run the hydraulic system with low water and little pressure, debris in the system may build on the interior walls and create blockages. Dehydration and excess proteins may be a contributing factor in arteriosclerosis.

Your Heart is a Pump - Maintain It

It is important to keep hydraulic pumps and their plumbing clear from the buildup of debris. To clean the debris off the walls of the hydraulic system, you would fill the system with fluid and run it at high pressure periodically. The occasional higher pressure will break off any debris that may have developed in the tiny pipes or on the walls of the larger pipes to keep the hydraulic system running smoothly. This is exactly what you need to do with your own heart and circulatory system.

Too often I see people out walking the same pace everyday. You need to raise your heart rate to in order to force open theses soft protein blockages and increase circulation. I believe exercising daily is extremely important. You can make your exercise more effective by bringing your heart rate close to the maximum heart rate for your age (no more than 85%). Do this by adding two 40 seconds sprints of walking faster in your walking, or other exercising every other day. The increase in blood flow is one of the most important steps in keeping your heart and vessels clear of plaque buildup.

Age	Target Heart Rate Zone 50% - 85%	Avg. Max. Heart Rate 100%
20	100-170 beats per minute	200 beats per minute
25	98-165 beats per minute	195 beats per minute
30	95-162 beats per minute	190 beats per minute
35	93-157 beats per minute	185 beats per minute
40	90-153 beats per minute	180 beats per minute
45	88-149 beats per minute	175 beats per minute
50	85-145 beats per minute	170 beats per minute
55	83-140 beats per minute	165 beats per minute
60	80-136 beats per minute	160 beats per minute
65	78-132 beats per minute	155 beats per minute
70	75-128 beats per minute	150 beats per minute
75	73-123 beats per minute	145 beats per minute
80	70-119 beats per minute	140 beats per minute

There are a few close variations regarding how to figure your maximum heart rate. These averages are only a guideline. Your maximum heart rate is 220 minus your age. The maximum heart rate for a fifty year old would be 170 (220-50=170). The figures in the previous chart are only averages. If you are taking medications for high blood pressure, check with your doctor. When beginning an exercise regime, start out slower, around 50% of your max heart rate.

Pump Your Lymph Nodes

Lymph nodes are throughout your body, especially in the creases. These creases include your ankles, bend of the knee, crease at the upper leg and pelvis, abdomen, elbow, underarms and neck. When you move and bend you are moving lymph by pressing the lymph vessels and nodes. The one crease where there are no lymph nodes is the wrists. Almost half of your lymph nodes are in your abdomen and the next most concentrated area is the neck. Exercises that utilize muscles in the abdomen and neck help increase lymph flow. Crunches are very good at putting pressure on the many lymph vessels and nodes in the abdomen and neck to help activate lymph. In a crunch, lie on the floor or your bed, cross your arms over your chest, bend your knees keeping your feet on the floor as you lift your head and shoulders slightly off the ground. As you do this the abdominal muscles, diaphragm and area of the cisterna chyli (major lymph junction by gall bladder) and neck are tightened, helping to propel lymph.

Make Your Exercise Convenient

Many individuals enjoy going to a gym to get their exercise. It becomes a part of their regular routine. Because we need to exercise daily, I purchased a treadmill along with some small hand weights so I can have the convenience of exercising at home whenever I have the time. Try to exercise at least 30 minutes a day for health maintenance and 60 minutes a day if you are trying to lose weight. Twice a week try to do a longer workout (45-60 minutes). If you're in a rush do at least 10-15 minutes of aerobics in your bedroom or on a treadmill, elliptical trainer or rebounder. Since you are doing a shorter workout after warming up, do your exercise at a faster pace or on an incline. Later in the day you can do another 15 minutes of exercise to total thirty minutes of exercise. If you don't help circulate blood through your tissues and organs on a daily basis you become filled with acidic waste, toxins and cellular debris. A simple 10 minute exercise routine I try and do daily is 2 sets of the following exercises 25 push ups, 100 crunches, 50 Jumping Jacks. Plus I do some walking, hiking, rebounding or biking a few days. Start slowly and increase your repetitions and endurance as your strength builds. The key, move your blood!

Rebounding Increases Circulation

Rebounding is a gentle and fun way to exercise. Rebounders are another piece of equipment every household should have. They are mini-trampolines that are around 40 inches across and a foot off the ground, some even fold in half for convenience. Rebounding is a good way to get a gentle whole body aerobic workout. There are many studies that show how rebounding helps to move lymph flow in the body. As you rebound, your tissues, blood and lymph vessels, organs, nerves, brain and spinal cord are all moving as you are jumping and impacting down on the rebounder. As you rebound up and down you increase lymph flow and blood circulation in the body. Almost everyone can exercise on a rebounder.

If you are not steady on your feet, it is advisable to order a stabilizing bar for additional support. My children now jump on the rebounder for fun instead of their beds. A sturdier, more durable rebounder with a "Soft-Bounce" is made in America by Needak Manufacturing and costs a few hundred dollars. You can also find rebounders with springs for seventy-five dollars at your local department store. Unfortunately, you get what you pay for and the less expensive rebounder is not made as well as the more costly ones. If you are overweight or have joint problems, you need a sturdier rebounder that can support your weight and a soft-bounce that will cushion your joints.

If you have pain, it is necessary that you find an exercise that doesn't increase your pain. Rebounders are very low impact, although if you have leg problems, recumbent stationary bicycles may support your body in a more comfortable sitting position. Find a few exercises that you can do comfortably and vary your workouts to avoid over use injuries.

In your exercise don't forget to raise and move your arms over your head. This may sound like an odd statement but when we walk or are riding a stationary bike we rarely move our arms overhead. One client who recently bought a rebounder said her arms began to swell after a few days of rebounding, so she stopped. I explained how the rebounding is activating lymph flow but her axilla (underarm) nodes were probably congested so the lymph was backing up into her arms. I asked her to show me how she was rebounding and her arms were either on the stabilization bar or hanging by her sides. I showed her how to self-activate her axilla nodes and how to do a few arm exercises like, alternating arms raised with fingers pointing to the ceiling or punching a make believe speed bag about head high. The idea is just too move your arms over your head more, it helps to open circulation in the major lymph drain in the left clavicle. Better still do the two-minute routine to self-activate your lymphatic system before you exercise, it will help open your circulation.

Good Posture – Stand and Sit Straight

Learning the benefits of good posture should begin as children. The body with its many vessels is similar to a complicated and sometimes minute plumbing system. When you slouch, whether sitting or standing you may be limiting your lymphatic system by putting extra pressure on tissues that may limit lymph flow and blood circulation. When manually mapping lymph flow in people who are standing straight; their lymph above the neck is flowing down to the major lymph vein beneath the clavicle. This is the way it should be flowing down, out of the neck and head. When I asked them to slouch a little, their lymph flow backs up into their neck and face. It stopped flowing changed direction and backed up. The lymphatic system is similar to a river, if you dam, crimp or block the lymphatic vessels that are meant to pick up the excess fluid and proteins in the tissues; fluid backs up in the tissues and organs. So stand and sit straight to keep your circulation moving.

Two Deep Breaths Could Change Your Life

We are a nation of what I call "Non-Breathers", meaning we take very shallow breaths. Look around you and watch people as they breathe. Most people tell me they are a shallow breather, especially when they are concentrating on a task, working on the computer or under stress. Your limited breathing habits are barely keeping you alive. Half of the lymph nodes are in your body are in your abdomen and neck. Deep breathing helps to push the lymph up the body to the heart to re-enter the blood supply. As your chest expands while deep breathing, your organs and lymph nodes in your abdomen, chest and neck are being compressed. This helps to decongest them and move the lymph and blood deeper into the tissues or organs.

Deep Breathing Exercises

Have you ever taken a few deep breaths consecutively? Try this exercise; take two to three deep breaths and then two regular breathes. Do this three times, make sure to take full deep breathes. Doesn't it feel good to have increased circulation in your tissues, bringing oxygenated blood to your cells. By just taking two or three sets of the two deep breaths, your extremities will tingle from the increased circulation. Be careful, you may get light headed or dizzy, so don't do breathing exercises while driving a car or operating any machinery.

For better health you need to take two deep breaths every few minutes throughout the day. If necessary, put signs up at home, at the office and in the car indicating "2 Deep Breaths" as a reminder. Make your children take two-three deep breaths often throughout the day, especially before bedtime. Deep breathing increases oxygen levels, superficial lymph flow, overall circulation and the ability of the body to clean itself.

In A Cast, Wheelchair Or Bed, Deep Breathe

If you are in a cast and are getting itchy inside the cast, don't try to scratch the itch. Do a few sets of 2-3 deep breaths, with two regular breathes in between and drink a couple of glasses of water over a few minutes. The deep breathing will move fluids through the limb affected by the cast, removing the toxins that were creating the itch. If you are in a wheelchair or bedridden deep breathing is especially important for you. Since you may not be getting enough movement in certain parts of your body, circulation can be impeded easily. When you aren't moving as much as you should be deep breathing and receiving lymphatic activation will help keep acid waste and proteins from building in your tissues and organs.

Water Can Make You Well

Drink water throughout the day, but especially thirty minutes before your meals, as well as at bedtime. Dr. F. Batmanghelidj believes dehydration is a major factor in disease that is being overlooked by the medical community. In his book "Your Many Cries For Water" the doctor writes of his experiences curing patients' ulcers and other problems with water. I believe Dr. Batmanghelidj has the right idea. Your body is made up of water, when you are even a little dehydrated your body's ability to function is compromised. In a two month old fetus, water accounts for 97% of the total body mass (TBM). In a newborn, water accounts for 72% of the TBM. In an average adult it's between 60 and 70% and in our seniors it's 50%. It seems that as we age we are becoming more dehydrated like a raisin in the sun.

You need water to thin your body fluids so they can flow deeper into your tissues and organs. Your cells are 90% water, brain tissue is 85% water, blood is approximately 90% water, lymph is 96% water and your cerebrospinal fluid is 98.5% water. If we are dehydrated, every system in your body can be affected by not having enough water. Many people drink tea, coffee, sodas, beer, wine and alcohol believing that the beverage at least has water in it. These do contain water but they act like a diuretic in the body making the need for water worse. I have met many people who drink no water and sustain on soda, coffee and beer thinking they are getting enough water. If you drink these beverages make sure you consume extra water and supplements. Dehydration concentrates and thickens the fluids of the body. The lymph could be thick similar to syrup, or with severe dehydration become like glue in your tissues or organs.

The fluids of the body need to be thin enough to pass through the cellular environment. We need ample amounts of mineralized water in order to stay healthy. Water in your body has many important roles. It carries nutrients and oxygen to cells, removes toxins, waste and proteins, it aids in digestion and the absorption of food, as well as regulating body temperature and blood circulation. Water plays an integral part in cushioning joints and protecting tissues and organs, including the brain and spinal cord, from trauma or infections like meningitis. Dr. Batmanghelidj recommends approximately two quarts of mineralized water a day, depending on your activity level.

Mineralized Water

It's important to know if your water contains adequate minerals. Check your drinking water with a pH test strip. If it tests acid, it is lacking many minerals.

For twelve years I carried five gallon jugs from the water store and thought I had healthy water. I had clean tasting water, but it wasn't as healthy as it could have been. Naturally mineralized water such as well water is alkaline. When water is treated chemically, and/or filtered by reverse osmosis, many of the minerals that help alkalize you are removed.

We need water but we need to drink mineralized water. Most bottled waters that say "drinking water" are filtered by reverse osmosis, which removes the minerals. Bottled water that says "Mountain Spring Water" is filtered but not using reverse osmosis, so it contains more minerals. You can use a single stage filter like the one attached to or in your refrigerator, or one you can screw right onto your sink faucet. These are only meant to remove some contaminants, like lead and chlorine while leaving more of the minerals. It is important to change your filter every six months, depending on your water use.

As a guide, you should try to consume ½ your body weight in ounces. If you are ill, take medication, work outside in the heat, do physical labor, or exercise you may need more water. If you drink soda, beer, or alcohol and smoke you should consume increased amounts of water. Don't wait until you are thirsty to have water, drink every half-hour. When you drink water take gulps not sips. You are trying to hydrate your whole body not just wet your lips. Check your urine to see if it is very dark or cloudy, which might mean you are dehydrated. Many of my patients tell me that they do drink plenty of water. Even though you think you drink enough water it may not be getting through to your deeper cells in the tissues. This is where exercise, massage and lymphatic activation can help open lymph flow so the deeper tissues can become hydrated.

Drinking adequate amounts of mineralized water may be one of the most important steps you can do to attain health.

CHAPTER EIGHTEEN

Step Four: Stress Reduction

Fight or Flight

When you are stressed, no matter how small the stress may be, physical changes occur in your body to prepare you for battle. The heart rate quickens, hormones start rushing, the body tightens, and your blood is retained more in the trunk of your body. This "fight or flight" response of the body is meant to last a short period of time until the threat or battle is over. Many individuals that we see at our wellness center have been trapped in a heightened stress response for many years, some for most of their lives. When you receive no relief from constant stress, the smallest amount of stress can create an extreme stress response. After long periods of sustained, uninterrupted stress, the body forgets how to relax. Circulation to the tissues becomes severely impeded, sleep becomes difficult, fatigue sets in, and your muscles tighten, further limiting circulation to your cells. After a while you aren't even aware of how tight your muscles have become. Stress is severely acid forming to the body. Most of us, even our children, live with enormous amounts of repeated stress on a daily basis. Stress is a known major contributing factor in most degenerative diseases.

Stress doesn't have to be life threatening to affect your health. Normal life is full of small stresses such as work deadlines, household duties, sitting in traffic, car problems, financial difficulties, health problems, dealing with children, homework, loss of a loved one and arguing with a spouse or friend. These stresses make your body react as if a physical threat had actually occurred. Some amount of stress will always be a part of your life. It is sustained and unmanaged stress that will kill you. To have a healthy life you need to learn how to manage the negative impact stress has on your health.

Massage: A Life-Enhancing Therapy

Hands have been used for thousands of years to alleviate pain, stress and to improve health. The practice of massage dates back to the Chinese in 3000 BC and almost every country in the world uses some type of hands-on therapy, like massage, to improve well-being. Each of them, in their own way, does one thing; activate the lymphatics to increase circulation. Hippocrates (460-377 BC) is considered the "Father of Medicine." According to Carl Sagan, renowned astronomer, Hippocrates was responsible for moving medicine into the "realm of science." You see, before Hippocrates, medicine was about superstitions.

Hippocrates was very aware of the benefits of massage and prescribed it for his patients. He used the Greek word anatripsis, which when translated means "to rub up." Hippocrates thought it best to stroke the extremities upward, rather than downward. He understood the positive effects of massage and wrote in his Corpus Hippocraticum (a collection of his writings) "The physician must be experienced in many things but assuredly in rubbing..." When you have pain from sciatica or a pinched nerve you have a choice to take medications or to receive massage or lymphatic activation to ease your pain. For thousands of years massage has been used to improve health. If you suffer from fatigue, pain or stress it is time you learn about the life enhancing benefits of massage therapy.

It is important to note that the idea of having to remove a poison from the body is not new. Aulus Cornelius Celsus, a Roman physician (42 BC-37 AD) followed Hippocrates' teachings. He wrote of rubbing the head to relieve headaches and rubbing the muscles to prevent paralysis. In trying to explain why friction (massage) creates positive results Celsus writes, "If we try to determine how these different results are produced (which is beyond the physician's realm) we see that they all consist in the removal of the noxious principle…Relaxation of the parts results after what made them hard is removed." Even around the time of Christ, physicians knew that there was a "noxious principle" in the body that makes you sick. That noxious principle that is hurting you is overly acidic and protein rich fluid in your tissues.

Massage Table in Every Home

Massage is so important to your health that I believe every household should have a massage table. In place of a massage table you can use a couch, bed or pillows on the floor. Just a few minutes two or three times a week, of some light pressure, rocking or stretching can change the way you feel. I believe it can lead to a positive change in an individual and family. When people receive massage they become less stressed and happier.

Most massage schools and colleges have classes for the non-professional to learn some basic anatomy, precautions and massage techniques. Even though my children are very young, when my wife or I have a tight neck or shoulders they volunteer to relax them by kneading our shoulder muscles. Massage is a wonderful way to learn how to touch in a positive way.

In our hurried society we have become starved for touch. Many people don't want to be touched and that's all right. This is also a trait common in children with autism. When your tissues are filled with acidic blood , your cells and tissues can become very sensitive. At first, being touched may seem uncomfortable, tickle or even hurt a little, as circulation in the tissues is changed the tissues relax and no longer hurt. Those who don't want to be touched are really the ones who need massage and other touch therapies the most.

I hope once you learn how important whole body circulation is to your physical and mental health you will try massage or other alternative therapy to activate the lymphatic system. I guarantee that after one or two sessions you will be a believer. If you are reluctant, many massage therapy centers offer a 15-minute chair massage that can relax the shoulders, neck, upper back and arms. Give it a try, your muscles may like it.

If you are ill, sensitive or apprehensive of having a massage CranioSacral Therapy (CST) is a really great way to start. In a CST session you are fully clothed and the therapist uses very light pressure on key areas of your body to increase your circulation. You will learn more about CranioSacral Therapy in the next chapter.

In my house we do shorter, fully clothed sessions, between 5–20 minutes a few times a week to activate the lymphatic system. Believe it or not, in 2-5 minutes you can get someone very relaxed and help increase circulation throughout their body. It only takes some gentle rocking and light pressure on the muscles to make a considerable difference. Even placing your hands gently on an area with pain for a few minutes will help to ease the pain. To make the massage even more effective, don't go with a full stomach, be well hydrated, have extra nutrients in your body, take some deep breaths and self-activate your lymphatic system after the massage.

Benefits of Massage

Relieves Pain and Stress
Relaxes Tense Muscles
Strengthens The Immune System
Helps Prevent Disease
Reduces Blood Pressure
Lowers The Heart Rate
Increases Circulation
Relieves Depression And Anxiety
Speeds The Healing Process
Helps Foster A Better Mind/Body Connection

What You Should Expect in a Massage

The most important thing you should expect to feel is comfortable. The massage therapy center should be clean and appealing. Try to find a center that fits your needs. Is it geared more for relaxation, or medical massage that can be more specific to your problem? If you haven't had one in a while, your first massage should be for increasing circulation through your body. A "Medium Deep Swedish Massage" is a great way to relax muscles and increase circulation with long flowing strokes called effleurage.

Most people go to a massage center and want a deep muscle massage as their first massage. It feels good when you are getting it, but the next day you feel beat up. This may discourage some people from getting another massage. At our old center we explained to our new patients that getting a deep massage at first may make them sore the next day, as stored toxins are released. Drinking extra water before and after a massage will help flush toxins out of the body.

Remember, you are paying for the massage. If anything is annoying to you, such as the music not being relaxing, the light being too bright, the massage too light or too hard or the therapist talks too much, you must let the massage therapist know. They want you to have a good experience so that you will feel comfortable and return. If you have a bad experience try another therapist until you find someone who you are comfortable with. In our center we book appointments every hour and 15 minutes. This gives the patient a full hour and allows them a few minutes to relax. The real secret of massage is that when it is done regularly, it has the ability to increase your circulation, relax your muscles, lower your risk of disease and enhance your quality of life.

Massage Increases Circulation

I am often asked, "How do I start a program to rid toxins from my body?" The best way to start is slowly with simple lifestyle changes, like eating a more alkaline diet, exercise, water and getting a few massages. A good road map is to follow the 5 Steps to balance the body and activate the lymphatic system. Many people try massage and expect miracles the first time. Even though many feel better after their first massage you can feel more sore or a little ill due to the waste being released. Try to have extra vitamins, minerals and water in your system to help buffer the excess acids that are released during a massage.

It may take many years for an individual to become tight and sick. You can get well, but it may take a few weeks or months of massage and then regular maintenance. In your first week of treatment, have one relaxing massage, in the second week have two massages two or three days apart. You may feel sore after your first massage as the extra released toxins create a healing crisis. In the third week, if you feel strong, try cleaning deeper into the tissues. I don't mean deeper as in deep muscle massage, as this can further traumatize tight tissue. You clean deeper into the tissues by increasing whole body circulation three days in a row. Do this by having a one-hour massage on three consecutive days. Each day as the therapist opens up congestion in the tissues, more toxins, acidic waste and proteins are removed. The idea is to enhance whole body circulation to change the overall cellular environment, rather than trying to work a few tight areas in the body. If you are on a budget do the same sequence of massages in half-hour sessions.

Regular Body Maintenance – Prevention is Key

No matter how healthy you are, you still accumulate waste and proteins in your body on a daily basis. Massage is an important step in keeping your tissues free of accumulating debris. How often you receive a massage really depends on what you can afford and how tight or sick you may be. Many people we see at our wellness center come in for a session every two to three weeks to manage their health. Some come in weekly because of they have stressful jobs or are sick and a massage allows them to function with less stress or pain.

We explain to our patients that their goal, once they are well, should be to maintain their wellness with a massage or other manual alternative therapies every two to four weeks. If you know a stressful situation is in the future, have a massage a few days prior to the event. Many people wait until after the stressful event when they are already stressed out, tight and have a migraine before scheduling a massage. This is too late, you are already congested.

Prevention is the key! To have vibrant health you have to learn to prevent the affects of stress from creating havoc in your body. Since you receive stress on a daily basis, you need to receive regular massage or alternative therapy to keep healthy.

Relax Someone's Shoulders

Since most of us have tight shoulders, very often I see a spouse or friend try to help relieve someone's tight shoulders but do it too hard. The first thing they do is squeeze the tops of the shoulders, called the trapezius (trap) muscles. This hurts! When the main drain of the lymph congests acidic fluid backs up into the trapezius and surrounding tissues. These muscles fill with toxic acidic fluid and become very sensitive. Next time you try to relax someone's shoulders, ask first and then stand behind them. Gently place your hands on their shoulders and traps, ask them to take two deep breaths. Now you can start to gently pump your fingers down to the nodes above the clavicles aiming under the clavicle bones about ten times. Then gently press your thumbs along the traps and shoulders starting by the base of the neck and moving an inch at a time toward the end of the shoulder. Gently press on each area of the traps and shoulders for a few seconds then repeat the whole process two or three times. Since you opened the lymph flow the light pressure will push acidic fluid out of the tissue, opening circulation and making the muscles less sensitive and tight.

Meditation: Think of Something That Makes You Happy

In an eight month long study at the Medical College of Georgia, 57 inner-city adolescents who practiced transcendental meditation for 15 minutes, twice a day, were able to increase the blood flow through their arteries by about 21%. The findings seem to suggest that people at risk for developing heart disease could use meditation as a way to maintain a healthy heart and better overall health. When you think of meditation many of you think of Transcendental Meditation (TM), where people will sometimes meditate for hours. Meditation, by its ability to relax you, can help increase your body's circulation and its ability to heal. Even just a few minutes, two or three times a day, will help to relax your body and mind. If you are sick, you should meditate on improving circulation in the affected area and health for 30 minutes, two or three times per day. When you meditate it doesn't have to be so formal, sitting with your legs crossed on the floor. Do it wherever you are comfortable, but won't fall asleep. Meditation can be a way to create a deeply, relaxed state of mind and body in a matter of minutes.

Try this easy meditation at home or even in your parked car, wherever you can find a few minutes of quiet. Remember a meditation is a state of mind. Take a few deep breaths, close your eyes and think of a person, place or thing that makes you happy, so happy you can't keep from smiling. This change in what you are thinking and feeling positively affects your whole body instantaneously. Find a comfortable straight sitting position and take two deep breaths. During the meditation try to include a few sets of two deep breaths. If you feel light headed, take more relaxed, slow breaths. If thoughts of work or errands that you have to do keep popping in your mind, just tell yourself that you don't want to think about that now and go back to your happy thought. Control your thoughts.

As you begin to visualize your happy thought begin to feel a sense of peace settle into your body and mind. Your image can be your child, family, spouse, a favorite memory, a vacation place, an ocean or mountain scene, it may even be a pet or a 57 Chevy. If you are thinking of an ocean scene, actually hear the waves crashing on the shore, feel the warmth of the sun on your face and body, feel the sand beneath your feet. As you take two deep breaths feel the ocean's spray hitting your face. Stay in this feeling of happiness and peace for a few minutes, remembering to take two deep breaths periodically. This meditation may only take a few minutes, but you just enjoyed a little mini-vacation from stress and increased your circulation.

Meditate On Your Life

If you meditated daily, even for a few minutes, you could change your life. As you continue to use meditation for relaxation, you can also use it as a tool to fine tune your life whether it is an upcoming business meeting, going over your golf swing or to help guide your life. When in a relaxed state of mind, meditate with reference to what you want to do with your life. Where do you want to be in six months or five years? Think about all aspects of your life, family, work, spirituality, play and health. When you meditate with what you want your life to be, you create a road map for your mind to follow. If you have no road map you have no direction. Start meditating on your roadmap to a better life today.

Being Able to Forgive

I mention this, because healing doesn't take place only in the physical body, it also takes place in the mind. You may have been traumatized or hurt by someone. Even though the physical scars may have healed, the emotional scars still linger and may be hurting you by limiting your circulation. When you hold onto the trauma (mental or physical) that happened to you, you are giving it control over your health. When you forgive someone, you aren't letting them off the hook; you are letting yourself off the hook. Instead of letting the trauma hurt you and cripple your life, let it empower you to never let it happen again. By forgiving and letting go you are taking back your life and health.

CHAPTER NINETEEN

Step Five: Manual Detoxification - The Real Key to Optimal Health

Your blood and lymph vessels are similar to an intricate, and sometimes minute, plumbing system with many twists and turns. In this plumbing system you have fluid, blood cells, acidic waste, hormones, fats, fibrin, cellular waste and minerals that can bind together to form small soft blockages. Whenever you move, exercise or deep breathe you help break up these little dams. Massage is a good way to break up debris in the tissues and help move some of it into the lymphatic vessels to be removed. Since we are overly acidic, our lymphatic system is compromised allowing some debris to remain in the tissues after a massage. This is similar to stirring up the water in your pool and not turning on the filter, the dirt will settle again.

In this chapter you will learn about a few life changing alternative therapies that dramatically increase lymph flow and blood circulation in the body. Therapies like CranioSacral Therapy, Visceral Manipulation, Lymph Drainage Therapy and Lymphatic Cellular Detox Massage activate the lymphatics and have the ability to work very specifically in the body, to enhance circulation where it is needed most, around the cells that make up your tissues, organs and central nervous system (brain, spinal cord and nerves). The most important step in your disease prevention plan should be regular lymphatic activation of the body, being specific to increase whole body circulation.

The doctors who developed these next few therapies are pioneers in manual medicine. Their techniques are literally helping hundreds of thousands of people around the world. Their decision to educate anyone who is licensed to touch the soft tissues of the body has spread their beneficial work across our nation and into many countries around the globe. Their goal was and still is to help as many as they can through educating other doctors, registered nurses, physical and occupational therapists and massage therapists to help others with their gentle work.

CranioSacral Therapy

CranioSacral Therapy (CST) is a light touch manual therapy that should be a part of everyone's body/mind maintenance. Your craniosacral system supports, nourishes and protects the brain and spinal cord. The dura mater is a tough membrane, it is the outermost layer of three membranes that surround the brain and spinal cord. The membranes should be able to glide or move as you move. The dura can become tight or restricted due to trauma, surgery, repeated epidurals or an overly acidic internal environment. This tightness in the dura can negatively affect your central nervous system. Your nerves begin at the spinal cord and pass through the dura to begin their journey throughout the body. If the dura is constricted from acidity, it can compress the beginning of your nerve, which can negatively affect the area specific to that nerve. Because of its ability to release restrictions in the dura, CranioSacral Therapy can gently affect far into the body to help release restrictions and increase circulation to accelerate healing.

We should start receiving CST from the day we are born. Sitting crunched up in the womb for nine months and surviving the birth process can stress a baby. A newborn session lasts approximately 15-30 minutes. In the session the newborn's craniosacral system is checked for restrictions (tight areas) and gently released. Older children or adult sessions are approximately 30-60 minutes. In CST we find restrictions in the tissues of the body with our hands and release them with very light pressure (the weight of a nickel). As the tissue releases from the therapist's light touch, circulation increases through the area. As fresh blood floods into the tissue, acidic fluid, waste, fibrin and other proteins that have caused you to feel tight, leave the tissue and the muscle relaxes.

Many patients have said they thought I had a heating pad under their back during a CST session. The heat they were feeling was their own blood finally flowing away from the core of their body and into their extremities and deeper into their tissues. During a session you will feel your tight muscles soften, as subtle releases occur to increase circulation. CranioSacral Therapy can be very specific, working with the cell or globally, including the entire body. It is one of the most grounding, stress reducing and totally beneficial therapies

I have ever experienced. After a CST session, patients often remark how they have never felt so relaxed in their life and later remark how well they slept after their CST session. I have experienced many of what you would call "miracles" with patients. For example, I often treat patients who have had years, sometimes decades, of debilitating pain. After only one or two one-hour sessions to specifically increase their circulation, a few called the next morning to say that they were pain free. These "miracles" were the result of increased circulation in toxic and tight tissues.

Contraindications of CranioSacral Therapy

CranioSacral Therapy is a light touch therapy that has profound effects on the body and brain. I believe everyone no matter how sick they may be, can benefit from a CranioSacral Therapy session. Some known contraindications are: recent bleeding in the cranium, intracranial aneurysm, recent skull fracture, and herniation of the medulla oblongata. Because of its ability to gently increase circulation, especially in the head include any health problems that may be negatively affected by any increased pressure in the head.

Visceral Manipulation

Your viscera are your internal organs, particularly those that are in the main trunk of the body. These organs include the intestines, stomach, liver, gall bladder, lungs, pancreas, spleen, heart, and reproductive organs. If you have experienced a fall, accident or severe emotional event, the trauma can be transferred to your organs and the ligaments and fascia that attach them to the body. The constricting effects of trauma, or an acidic environment, limit the organs' circulation and its ability to function.

Your organs are not separated into neat little compartments, they are pressed against each other or gliding over one another. If one organ is restricted, it could be affecting the other organs and surrounding tissue. The therapist who practices visceral manipulation uses very light specific stretches to release the tight tissue and ligaments surrounding the organ. This increases mobility and fluid circulation in the organ and its surrounding tissues. I often feel hard tissues actually soften in my hand after a few gentle stretches of the soft tissue and fascia. Acidic and hard tissues and organs don't allow for optimal circulation.

Contraindications of Visceral Manipulation

Visceral manipulation is very gentle, but when working with the viscera you have to use your common sense. If tissues around an organ are painful to the touch or hot and inflamed, avoid treating until the inflammation or pain is under control. Any abnormal, sudden or acute pain is a contraindication for visceral work. Also include any tumor or mass, fevers, cancer, abdominal aortic aneurysm, duodenal ulcers, gallstones, pregnancy, IUDs, and fractures as contraindications for visceral work.

Lymph Drainage Therapy

A proper functioning lymphatic system is critical in keeping us free of infection and disease. The lymphatic system is connected to every system in the body, including the craniosacral and visceral systems. If the lymphatic system is slowed or malfunctioning, it could be detrimental to your health. Lymph Drainage Therapy (LDT) is very specific in enhancing lymph flow and blood circulation through the tissues, including the organs. When lymph flow is increased in the body it is similar to releasing water from a dam. The increased fluid flow through the tissues can begin to remove accumulated debris such as acidic waste, fibrin, hormones and cholesterol that may have accumulated in the vessel or tissue. When you improve lymph flow you improve detoxification in the body.

Mapping Lymph Flow

In Lymph Drainage Therapy we monitor the superficial and deep lymph flow anywhere in the body. Lymph drainage therapists use their hands to map lymph flow through the tissues. When they find areas of congestion, they first enhance lymph flow to that area. The therapist then uses specific soft tissue techniques, to gently breakup fibrosis in the area. LDT is then used to enhance the lymph flow through the tissues to help evacuate debris. Lymph Drainage Therapy is very effective at removing acidic waste, toxins and excess proteins from around the cells. This increases circulation, improves the pH around the cells and improves your health.

Cancer and Lymph Activation

When circulation becomes stagnant in an area within your tissues, organs or bones, the disease process can begin. In our society there is a misconception that massage or manual therapies may spread cancer. To this date there is no real scientific research that has shown that manual therapies, such as massage or manual lymph drainage, spread cancer. Professor M. Foldi, M.D. of

Germany was an early lymph therapist and researcher. He writes, "The possibility of inducing malignant modifications with manual (lymph) treatment has been excluded."

In cancer treatment you are told to exercise which also activates the lymphatic system. So if you can exercise you can receive lymphatic activation. Increasing lymph flow does not spread cancer, it helps to build the immune response. Increasing circulation to increase oxygen and nutrient levels and waste removal in the tissues is very important in any disease, especially cancer. **Do not have any bodywork or perform self-lymphatic activation a few days before or after a chemotherapy or radiation treatment.**

Contraindications of Lymph Drainage Therapy

LDT is a very gentle therapy that has a powerful effect on the fluid systems of the body. A general rule of thumb in LDT is that if the patient can climb up a flight of steps without becoming winded, they can handle an LDT session. Contraindications include: serious circulatory problems (i.e., blood clots and obstructions in the veins), acute infections, high fevers, major cardiac problems (i.e., acute angina pectoris and recent heart attack), active bleeding, and absence of urination.

Lymphatic Cellular Detox Massage

Toxins are everywhere, in the air we breathe, in the water we drink and the food we eat. There is no avoiding them unless you want to live in a bubble. Our homes are sealed tightly to keep the outside from coming in. This also traps the air within our homes, which is filled with toxic fumes from carpets, furniture, paints, air fresheners, cleaners, and pesticides. The most important step in regaining your health is removing these toxins from your body on a regular basis so they can't accumulate. The most efficient way to rid the body of toxins is through lymphatic activation, which manually increases fluid circulation and detoxification through your tissues.

CranioSacral Therapy, Visceral Manipulation and Lymph Drainage Therapy open circulation and detox specific parts of the body. Each therapy individually is extremely powerful. By combining the ideas of the three therapies into a specific routine to increase whole body circulation, the work becomes even more powerful. After learning about tissue acidosis, I started researching the most efficient way to manually remove acidic waste, toxins, fibrin, and other proteins from our tissues. Almost two years later, and after hundreds of sessions, I developed "Lymphatic Cellular Detox Massage." It is the first manual detoxification therapy in North America that, in one hour, specifically increases circulation through the tissues, organs, brain, spinal cord, and nerves to help remove acidic waste and excess proteins. It opens microcirculation deep in the spaces around your cells.

Remember, we "live and die at the cellular level." Patients are always remarking how they feel tingling in their extremities during the first session of Lymphatic Cellular Detox Massage. This tingling is due to increased circulation to the starved cells. Many of the patients I see have tried eating healthier, using nutritional supplements and herbs, as well as receiving many manual alternative therapies to diminish their pain or stress, sometimes with minimal results. Patients feel a difference after lymphatic activation because it gets to the root of their problem, which is lack of circulation and resulting buildup of acidic waste in and around their cells.

Contraindications for Lymphatic Cellular Detox Massage

Everyone can benefit from Cellular Detoxification Massage. If you are ill or pregnant, consult with your doctor. Since Cellular Detoxification Therapy is based on a combination of the three therapies, follow all aforementioned contraindications.

Patient Profile: Marlene J.

When Marlene first walked into our wellness center she was dressed all in black. You could see that her left arm and shoulder were tight as she held her arm securely against her body. Her left leg dragged a little behind as she walked to a chair. Her face looked emotionless, as if she had already given up. My office manager gave me the new patient information sheet that Marlene was required to fill out. It was untouched except for her name across the top. Marlene was in a dark mood that day. She said that she had always been a vibrant person, but had recently resigned herself to the fact that there was no hope for her declining health.

Marlene's health problems had started as a young child with low back pain and kidney problems. As a preteen she had severe acne and at fourteen she received outlawed radiation treatments on her face for her acne. As a teenager her chronic back problems almost crippled her. As an adult she had bad allergies, sinus infections, bronchitis, dry-itchy skin, hemorrhoids, continued back, hip and neck tightness and several severe colds per year. Unhappy with having to take medications and still feeling sick, Marlene decided to take charge of her life and become more health conscious. She became a vegetarian, studied Homeopathy, herbs, vitamins and minerals. She had tried separate sessions of CranioSacral Therapy and Lymph Drainage Therapy over the years and even became a massage therapist. She had spent years doing all the right things to promote health but her health just continued to deteriorate.

Marlene began having severe pain in her left arm and left leg which would last for several hours. These episodes continued for several weeks until Marlene thought she was having a heart attack, or possibly a stroke, and finally went to the emergency room. After being admitted and examined further she was found to have been suffering from Transient Ischemic Attacks (TIA). TIA's are little strokes in the brain, which are warning signals for an oncoming, more serious stroke. She was prescribed a baby aspirin per day and given a prescription for cholesterol lowering drugs, which she did not fill.

Marlene was becoming worse. She became sensitive to many chemicals. Her thinking was becoming foggy and she had no center of gravity, which caused her to be unsteady on her feet. Marlene was always tired, had severe mood swings and fought depression. Her doctor had recently found two or three small benign masses in her face and neck that had to be removed. She knew she was getting worse when she could no longer add numbers in her head. She found out that she was having symptoms of Normal Pressure Hydrocephalus (NPH), which can occur in individuals of any age, but is most common in seniors. It is an excessive accumulation of fluid (CSF) in the brain that may result from a subarachnoid hemorrhage, head trauma, complications of surgery, infection or a tumor. It is important to note that many people who develop NPH have none of these complications, in these cases there is no known cause. One possible reason for excess fluid on the brain is a malfunctioning lymphatic system due to acidity and protein proliferation.

When I first monitored Marlene's lymph flow, her whole lymphatic system was very congested, more so in her shoulders, neck, face and head, which can limit flow to her brain. Her lymph fluid was flowing poorly and in the opposite direction, filling the tissues with excess fluid and proteins. Fifteen minutes into a combined session of CranioSacral Therapy and Lymph Drainage Therapy, Marlene's lymph flow was moving better. I had one hand under the base of her neck and shoulders and one hand resting gently on her upper chest, allowing her upper body, neck and head to release and have increased circulation. As I held this position for a few minutes Marlene said she was beginning to feel tingling in her left leg.

I explained how complete blood circulation is dependent on lymph flow and that the main lymph drain is by your left clavicle at the base of the neck. When we gently hold, open or drain the clavicle nodes, it is similar to opening a clogged drain. This increased lymph flow can help increase blood flow throughout the body. The tingling she experienced in her leg was the result of waste removal and increased blood flow through her muscles, bringing oxygen and nutrition to her cells. She actually got emotional and excited while talking with me about feeling this tingling in her leg. Understand, she had given up all hope. To her this tingling was renewed hope. After the session, Marlene said she felt looser and more alive than she had felt in a long time. She repeatedly spoke about having hope again.

The next morning she felt tired, achy and congested, as if she were getting the flu, "The Healing Crisis." I could already notice a loosening in her left arm and leg as she walked into the office for her second session. Marlene had a smile on her face and she was more jovial. By the second week, after five sessions, Marlene was a different woman. Her constricted arm and leg were back to normal and she was able to think again, even able to add numbers in her head. She is wearing bright colors instead of the black she often wore. She has a new bounce in her step and is happy again.

Marlene is a perfect example of individuals who try everything but their health continues to fade. She had tried many different dietary and manual therapies but to little avail. When we activated her lymph flow, especially in her organs and craniosacral system in a specific manner, it allowed the body to clean and nourish itself. In less than two to three weeks Marlene was happy and whole again. Marlene understands the need for maintenance sessions and there are days that she comes in and says her lymph feels all clogged up. She comes in every three or four weeks and occasionally she will do two consecutive sessions to clean deeper into her tissues. Marlene is maintaining well because she understands the importance of an 80% alkaline and 20% acid diet, nutritional supplementation, daily exercise, stress reduction and lymphatic activation. Marlene has taken responsibility for balancing her life for improved health.

CHAPTER TWENTY

Self–Help Techniques

Self-Lymphatic Activation

The lymphatic system is connected to every system in the body, when congested it can lead to a backup of fluid and waste anywhere in the body. This slow or stagnant fluid goes through chemical changes becoming more acidic and toxic from added cellular metabolic waste and debris. Tight muscles, inflammation, pain, infection, swelling, premature aging, cysts, cancer and many other health problems can occur if this congestion is left unchecked and not treated. If you were to manually move your own lymph on a daily basis you could lose weight have less headaches and acid reflux, more energy, improved health and age more gracefully with an intact mind.

Self-Activate the Lymph in Your Nodes and Tissues Daily

When you activate the lymph in a tissue or organ you are actually increasing and completing blood circulation. You should use a soft, gentle sweep of the skin to increase the lymph flow in the tissues. When you drain a tissue it's best to start learning by using one long soft sweep from the end of an extremity to its main nodes also called mother nodes. When a group of nodes are being activated use a soft, gentle pump into the body and then finish the pump towards the direction of the heart. Try to create a wave like motion as you gently compress the area of the nodes. As you become more proficient in self-lymphatic activation, you can use five gentle stretches of the skin every 6–8 inches starting at the main lymph nodes and working to the end of the extremity and back to the nodes. Before enhancing your lymph flow, you need to open the major lymph nodes of the area you are working on. Opening the mother nodes will begin to increase circulation throughout the body.

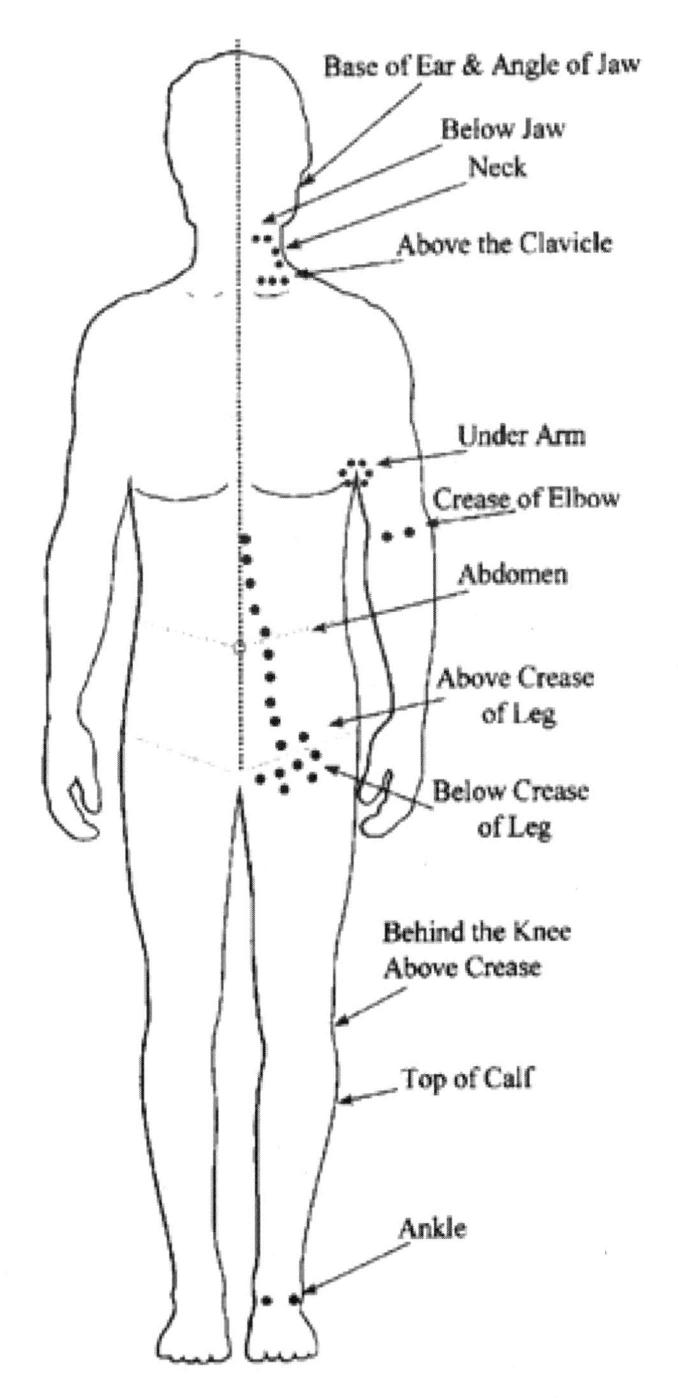

Fig. 20.01 Lymph nodes are found in many folds of the body. As you bend and move, you put pressure on many of these areas helping to move lymph.

Location of Main Lymph Nodes

By manually pumping or draining certain parts of your body you can self-activate your lymphatic system. (Fig. 20.01) The main area of nodes in the body are at the base of the neck above the clavicles (supraclavicular nodes), underarms (axilla nodes), cisterna chyli (three vessels by the gall bladder), crease at the top of the leg (inguinal nodes), crease behind the knee (popliteal nodes) and sides of the ankle (malleolar nodes).

After a few weeks of awkwardness, you will eventually become very proficient in activating your lymph and lymph nodes. It will become a routine you will be able to utilize to increase circulation in a few minutes, in order to ease pain or congestion in any area of your body. Find a lymph drainage therapist in your area who can further help you improve your circulation.

Caution: Never try to specifically increase circulation during high fevers, active infections, active bleeding and acute life-threatening illnesses, seek medical attention. Increasing circulation would create excess waste in the system and make the fever or infection worse, "the healing crisis." Wait a day or two until the fever has broken or until the infection is under medical control.

The Shoulder Shuffle

Any time you feel tight in your shoulders or neck, try this self-help technique to increase circulation and alleviate muscle tension in the neck and shoulders. Raise one shoulder towards your ear and then put it down, keep your head straight while raising your shoulder. Repeat raising the other shoulder to the ear. Do four or five repetitions of alternating shoulder raises in a quick rhythm. This action relaxes the tissues and vessels and opens circulation in the area of the base of the neck and main lymphatic drain.

1. The Main Lymph Drain Under the Left Clavicle

The main drain of the lymphatic system is a lymph vessel/vein connection; it is located under the left clavicle, where the thoracic duct meets the left subclavian vein. A very small percentage of individuals will have the main drain located on the right side, located under the right clavicle. (Fig 20.02) It is at this connection in the left shoulder that a blockage can easily occur and affect other parts of the body. A tight back, chest or shoulders, as well as a small blockage or buildup of debris in this area of the main drain, can interfere with lymph flow throughout the body, similar to damming a river. You can help to keep this main

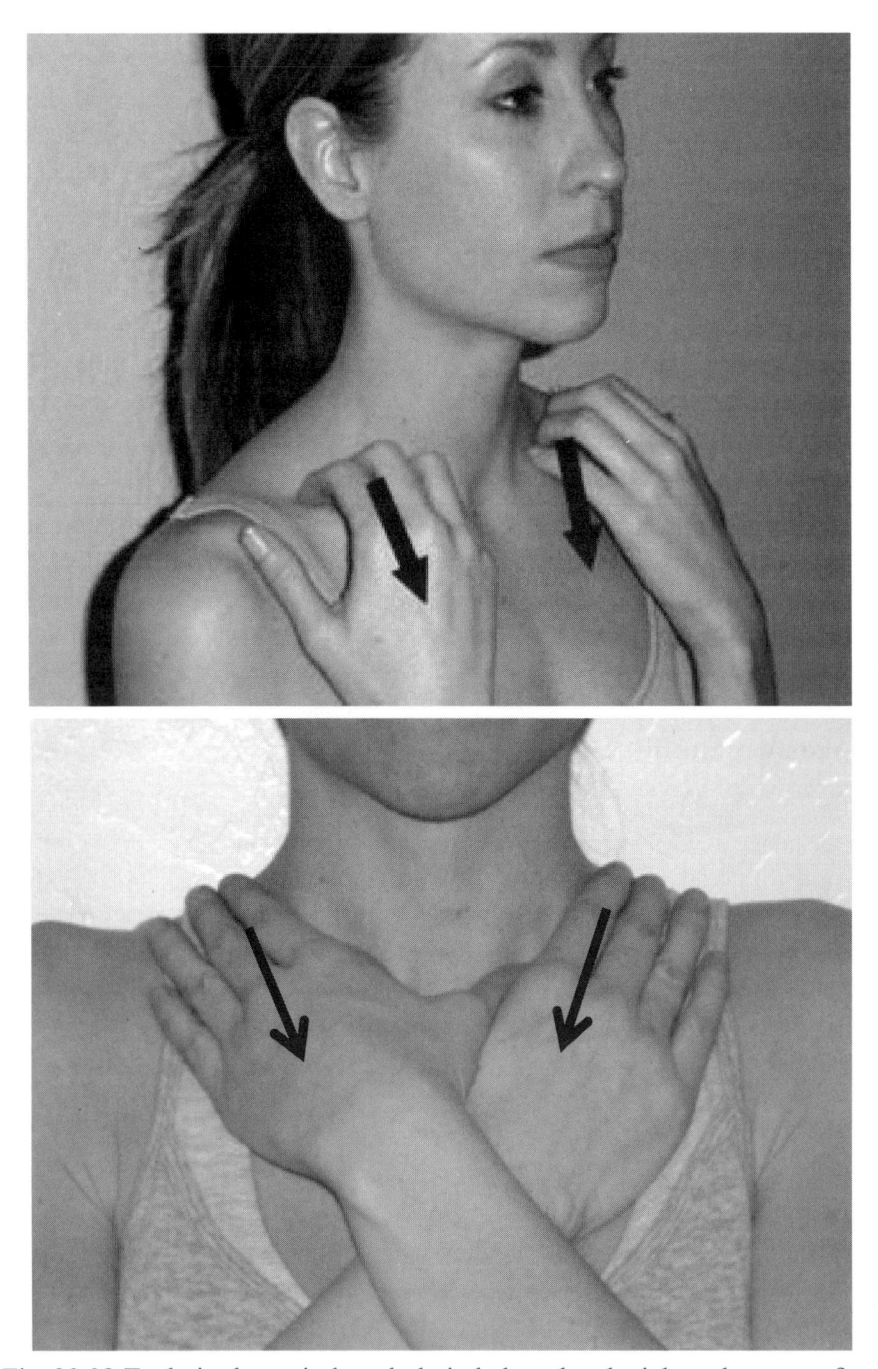

Fig. 20.02 To drain the main lymph drain below the clavicles, place your fingers behind the clavicles or cross arms and place fingers on the soft triangle above clavicles and gently pump aiming down under the clavicles, towards the heart.

lymph drain area open by gently pumping or moving and stretching your neck, shoulders and stretching your arms over your head.

Now that you have opened circulation in the neck area by alternately raising your shoulders to your ear a few times you are ready to manually drain the main lymph drain. This drain is located below the soft triangle formed by your left shoulder, neck and clavicle bone. This triangle is called the supraclavicular fossa and contains lymph nodes. Gently pumping these nodes above the clavicle bones (supraclavicular nodes) down; helps to increase lymph flow in the main lymph/vein connection and other parts of the body. To find and drain this soft triangle, raise your bent left elbow up even with your ear this. The soft triangular indentation formed where your shoulder, neck and clavicle meet, is where the supraclavicular nodes are located.

To drain this area you can cross or uncross your arms and place your fingers above the clavicle bones in the soft triangle. Place the pads of three fingers gently onto the indentation of the soft triangle and gently pump this area down, aiming under the clavicle bone towards your heart. You are trying to create a slow rhythmic wave with your gentle pumping to increase circulation through the nodes and lymph-vein connection improving lymph flow. As you end your pump and begin to return to your original location, where you started the pump, try to release pressure on the skin on your upwards movement. This keeps fluid from being pulled back up into the area.

Gently pump the nodes above the clavicle downward 5 to 10 times, one to two times per day. Do the right and left nodes above the clavicle on either side of the base of the neck. Remember to take two deep breaths often while draining your lymphatic system. Try to create a slow rhythmic wave as you pump down in the direction of the heart.

Drain Your Neck and Face

The lymph in your neck and face drains down into the nodes and vessels above your clavicles (supraclavicular nodes) on either side of your neck. Consequently, before you drain the neck or any part of the body you should always first drain the nodes above the clavicles down to the heart.

When lymph in the neck and face back up, many problems can arise; acne, rosacea, thyroid problems, tight neck, headaches, migraines, sore throat, earaches, fluid congestion in ear, ringing in ears, sinus problems, bulbous nose, eye allergies, dry eyes, bags under the eyes, dry mouth, sensitive teeth, inability to think clearly, hair loss, swollen lymph nodes and TMJ pain. Draining your neck and face daily would increase circulation and help most of the above problems.

2. Neck

To drain the neck, place both hands on the opposite sides of your neck and stretch the skin down. (Fig. 20.03) To make sure you have the right hand positions, place your hands on your throat as though you are going to choke yourself with both hands. Loosen your grasp on the neck; the pads of your fingers should be on the sides of your neck. Gently stretch the skin beneath your finger pads down towards the nodes above the clavicle. Don't slide on the skin with your fingers, contact the skin and stretch the skin down.

Firmly but softly place your fingers to the skin and gently stretch the skin down, aiming under the clavicle bone. At the end of the stretch always release your hand pressure on the skin slightly as you return to your original position to avoid pulling fluid back up into the area.

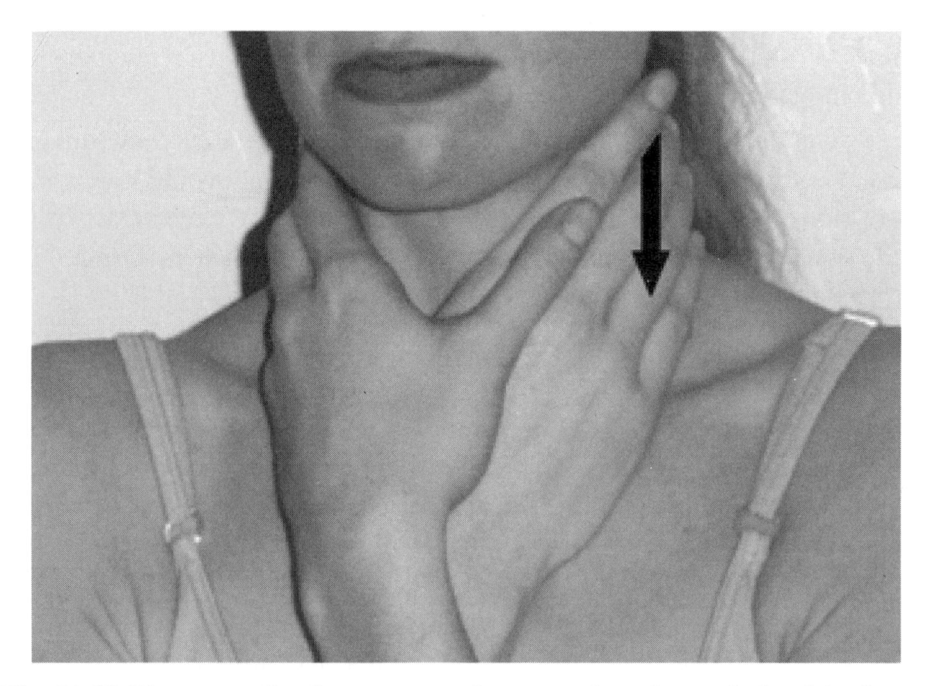

Fig. 20.03 Place your flat fingers around your neck and stretch the skin down, aiming under the clavicles, to the center of the chest.

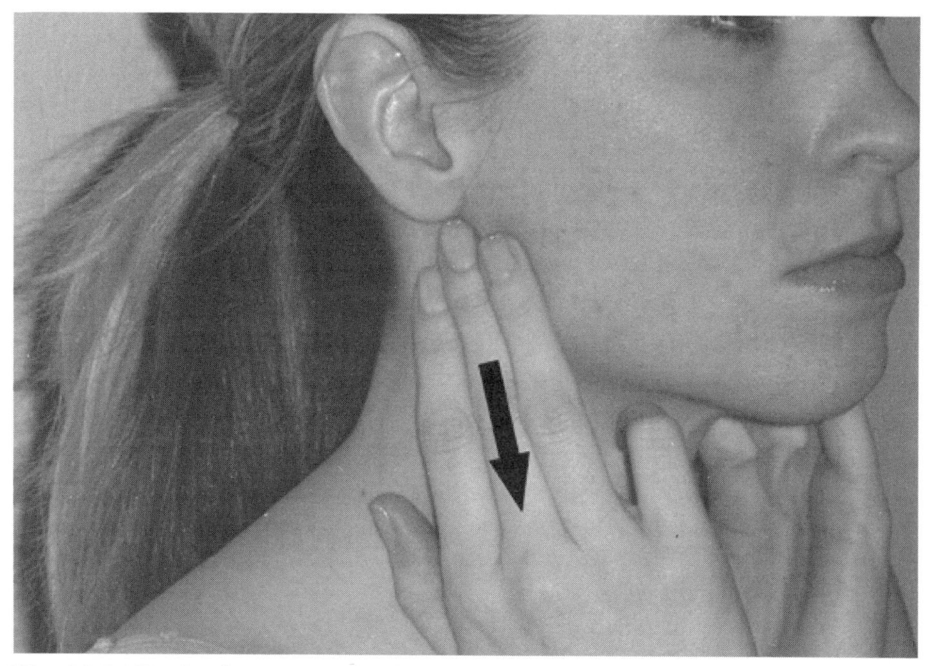

Fig. 20.04 Drain the water wheel (nodes below the ear) down to the clavicles.

3. Water Wheel

The water wheel is a cluster of nodes that sit at the base of each ear, between the jaw and neck. It is made up of the jugulodigastric nodes and the superior deep cervical nodes. These are very important nodes to drain in order to keep the lymph in the neck, face and head flowing. Place three fingers at the base of the ear, pointing up. (Fig. 20.04)

Your middle finger should be in the little channel formed between the jaw and the neck. Gently stretch the skin down with all three fingers. If you have ear and other health problems above your clavicles, open the nodes above the clavicles, drain the neck and then drain the water wheel down into the neck, a few times throughout the day.

4. Nodes Below Your Jaw

Your lymph nodes and salivary glands can become congested and swell when you have an infection or are sick. Many of you have felt the little nodules below your jaw. They are the submandibular lymph nodes and submandibular glands (below the jaw). Our focus is to activate the nodes and lymph vessels in the area, which will help increase circulation and benefit the glands. The nodes below the jaw drain from the center of the chin to below the ear, or more specifically to the water wheel. An easy way to activate them is by using your softened fists to drain the area. (Fig. 20.05)

Make fists with your hands and raise them to either side of your chin. Soften your fists and rest your jaw on the platform made from your bent fingers. Use your bent fingers to gently sweep the soft tissue beneath your jaw towards the water wheel (towards your ear). Start at the chin and gently sweep under the jaw up to the base of the ear.

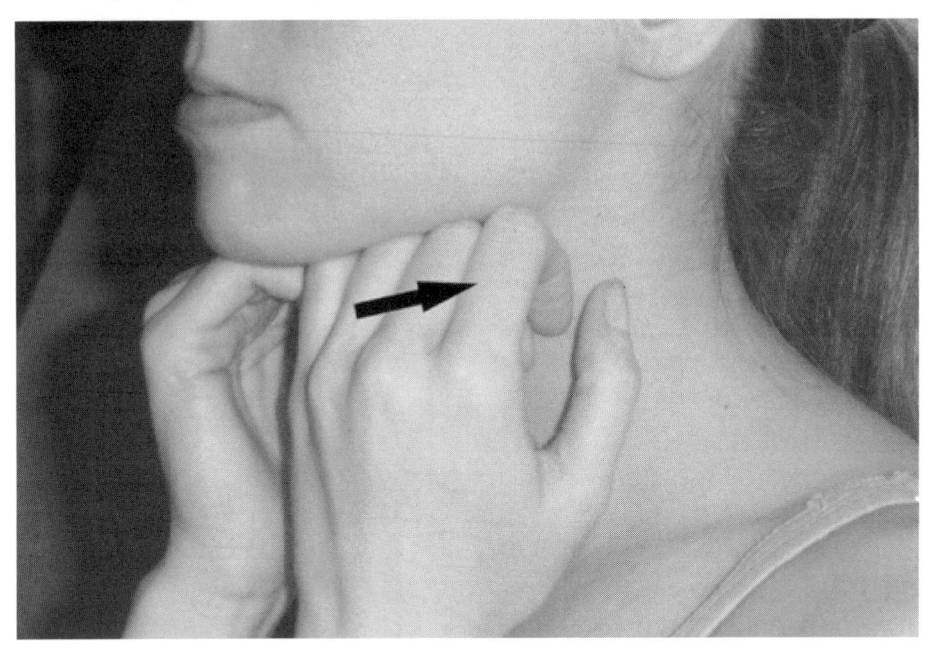

Fig. 20.05 Use your soft fists as a platform to drain the nodes below the jaw. Sweep the soft tissue behind the jaw from the center of the chin to the base of the ear.

5. Cone of the Face

The face has two separate pathways for superficial lymph flow. The first area to be drained is the cone of the face (Fig. 13.01). To find the cone of the face, draw an imaginary line from between your eyebrows above your nose, to just below the angle of your jaw. Lymph inside the cone of the face drains down to the submandibular nodes, below the jaw.

An easy way to drain the cone of the face is by placing your middle fingers along your nose, touching the center of the eyebrows. (Fig. 20.06) The only fingers touching the side of the nose and face are the middle fingers. Use the whole middle finger to make contact with the skin. Gently slide the fingers down from the eyebrows along the nose. As your middle fingers pass the tip of your nose, allow your ring and index fingers to join the middle fingers to make contact with the skin and slide straight down over the lips to the jaw.

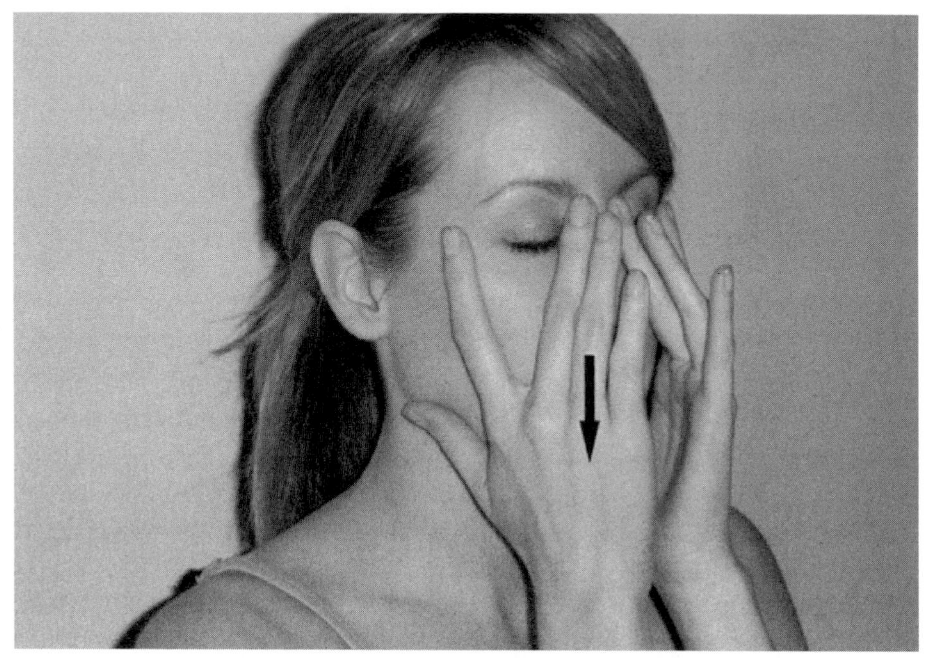

Fig. 20.06 Drain the cone of the face from the center of the eyebrows down to the nodes below the jaw.

6. Parotid Nodes

The next area of the face to be drained is outside the cone of the face. This area includes the sides of the face, under the eyes, temples, forehead and the front half of the top and sides of your head.

Outside the cone of the face drains to the parotid nodes, which are located near the parotid glands just below your ear, near the angle of your jaw. Place your flat fingers over the angle of the jaw. (Fig. 20.07) Your index fingers should be by the water wheel (by the base of the ear). Gently pump and stretch your flat fingers towards the base of the ear.

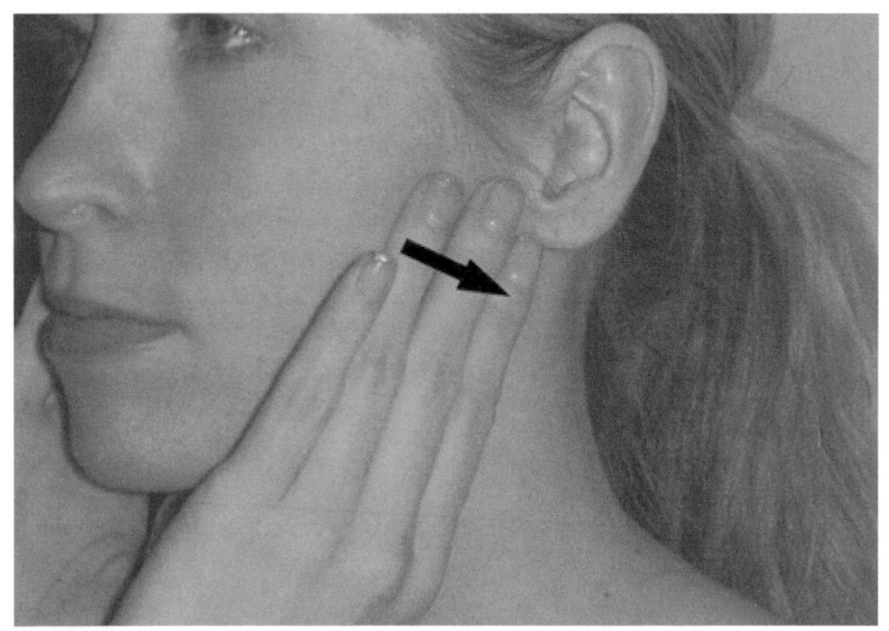

Fig. 20.07 Drain your parotid nodes by placing your flat fingers over the angle of the jaw and gently pump into the base of the ear.

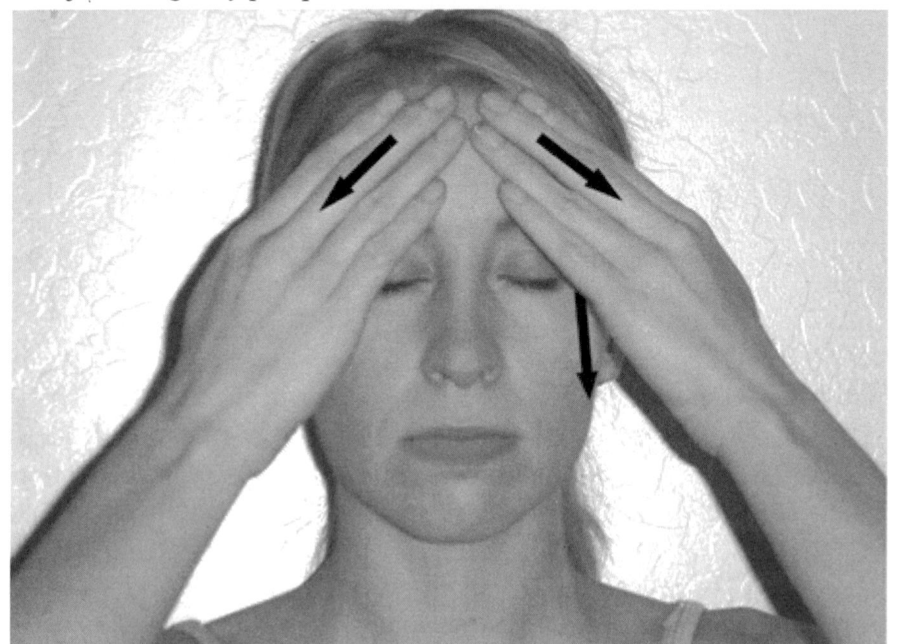

Fig. 20.08 Drain your forehead, scalp and temples by sweeping your flat fingers from the center of your forehead, over the temples to your parotid nodes (angle of the jaw), aiming at the base of your ear.

7. Forehead to Parotid Nodes

After opening the parotid nodes (by the angle of the jaw) place your flat fingers to each side of the center of the forehead and sweep down over the temples to the parotid nodes (below the ear at the angle of the jaw). (Fig. 20.08) If you have TMJ pain or dysfunction, open this area often throughout the day. After sweeping the forehead to the ear sweep from the top middle of the head and hairline down to the temples and then to the parotid nodes at the base of the ear. This helps thinning hair by increasing circulation to the roots of your hair.

8. Axilla Nodes

The axilla nodes are in your underarm. You can drain these nodes by using the fingers of the opposite hand to pump gently but deeply into the underarm. (Fig. 20.09) Place the pads of four flat fingers across the underarm and rhythmically pump deep into the underarm aiming slightly up and towards the center of the chest. The action should feel like a rhythmic wave, not a squeeze. This area can become dry and feel as if dried crystals are in the tissue of the underarm. After a few lymph drainage therapy sessions, the tissue becomes hydrated and the crystals dissolve. Self-lymphatic activation may take a few weeks, but you will see good results if you give it the time.

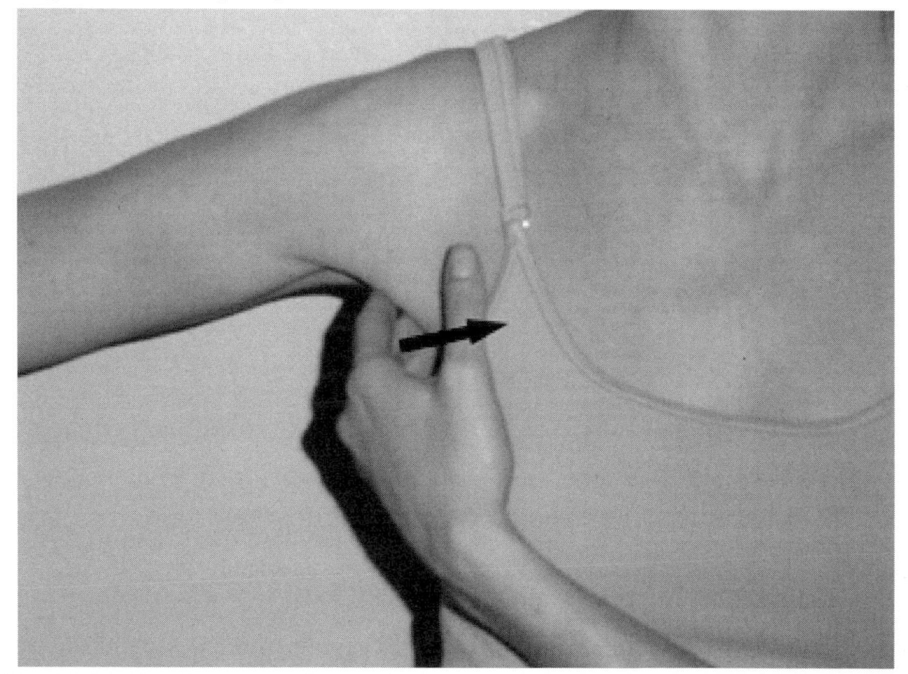

Fig. 20.09 Gently, pump deeply into the underarm, aiming up and in, towards the center of the chest.

Congested axilla nodes may lead to breast swelling, breast cysts, nipple discharge, breasts on men, breast pain, frozen shoulder syndrome, rotator cuff problems, carpal tunnel syndrome, ganglion cysts, arm swelling, tennis elbow, arthritis in the fingers and pain or numbness in the hand or fingers.

9. Drain Arm

If you wanted to activate the lymph in your left hand and arm, you would raise your left arm up straight out in front of you, slightly above your heart with your palm facing down. (Fig. 20.10) If you can't raise your arm easily, support it with a pillow or two on your lap. Place the flat fingers of your right hand up to the fingers of your left hand. With no added pressure slowly slide the pads of your fingers up the arm into the underarm. Stay on the inside (soft part) of the arm and as you reach the underarm pump gently but deeply towards your heart.

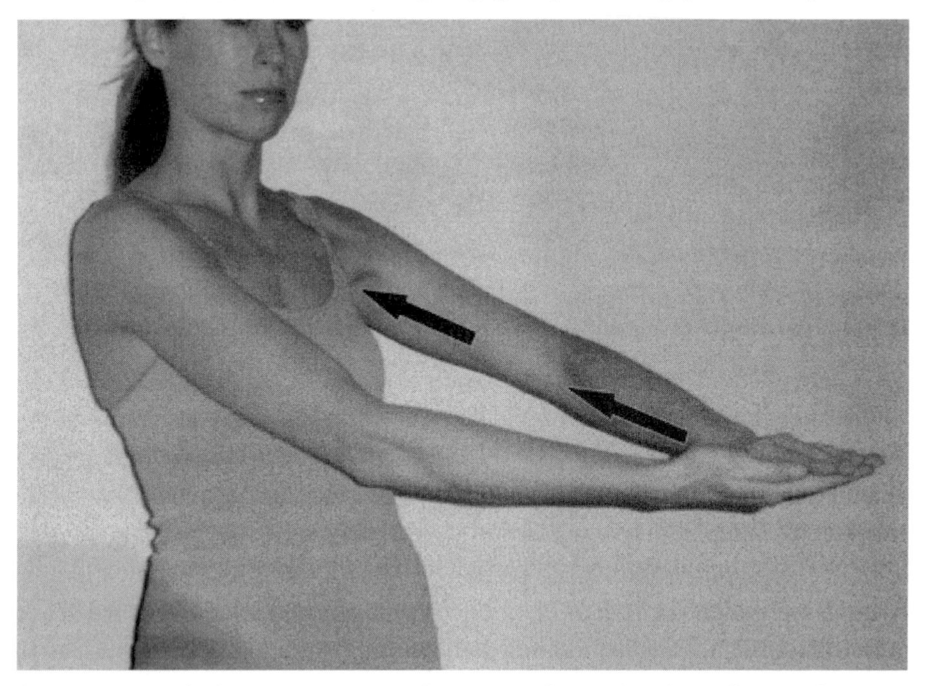

Fig. 20.10 To drain your arm gently sweep from the tips of your fingers up along the inside of the arm, ending deeply into the underarm.

10. An Important Lymph Drain – Cisterna Chyli

The cisterna chyli is where the main lymphatic vessels (three vessels) that drain the legs, abdomen and pelvis, converge into one vessel. These three vessels merge to become the thoracic duct, which begins by the gall bladder and right rib cage and ends in a main vein before the heart. Often with clients who have circulation problems in their legs, I only have to open their cisterna chyli to feel an immediate positive change in the lymph flow in their legs. This indicates to me that the problems in the legs are compounded by the congested cisterna chyli, which is situated close to the liver, gall bladder and diaphragm.

I believe the backup of toxic lymph in the area of the cisterna chyli can be the cause of many of our unexplained pains in the gall bladder area. Many people who suffer with pain in this area end up having their gall bladder removed, even though the organ may have only been congested. The gall bladder is almost completely encapsulated by lymph vessels. An overly acidic and protein filled gall bladder can become very constricted and painful.

Drain the cisterna chyli by placing your left hand under your right rib cage. The heel of your hand is by the midline of your body, your index finger follows the angle of the ribs and your thumb is on the inside of the ribs. (Fig. 20.11) Then place your right hand over your left hand and rhythmically pump in and down with both hands 3-5 times to open congestion in this area then pump in and up towards the center of your chest 5-10 times. Aim your pumps up along the rib cage then up towards the heart.

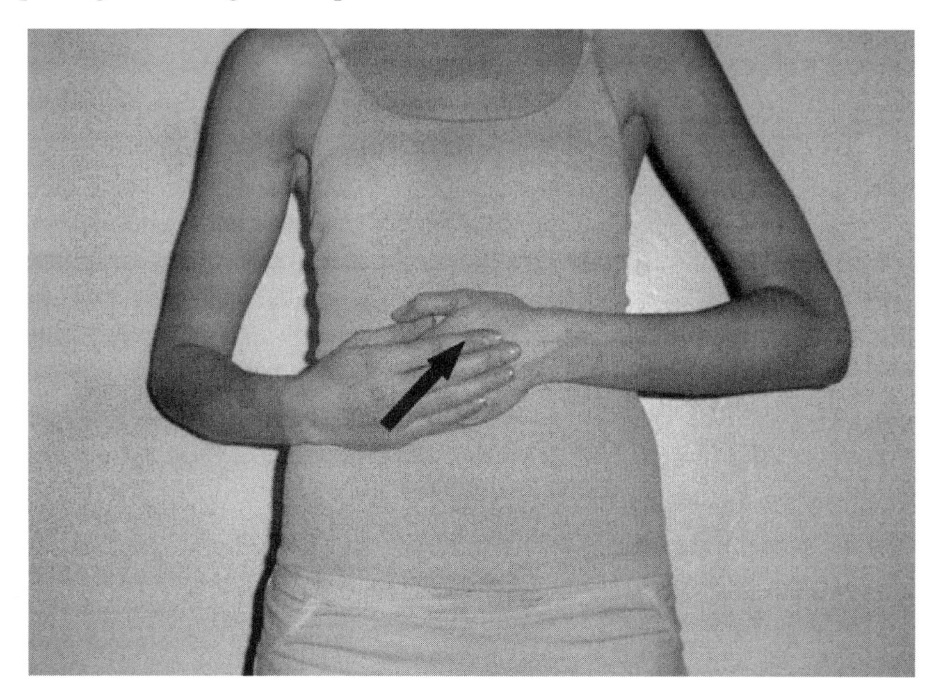

Fig. 20.11 Use both hands below your right rib cage and gall bladder to drain the cisterna chyli down 3-5 times, then up and towards the heart 5-10 times.

This is a group of lymph vessels that can congest easily. If you have problems with your legs, abdomen, digestion, pelvis, prostate or reproductive organs this is an important place to drain.

11. Drain the Upper and Lower Abdomen

Almost half of your lymph nodes are in your abdomen so this is an important place to drain. Very often the cisterna chyli can become congested and allow fluid and proteins to build in the small intestine, colon, rectum and cavity of the stomach. Place one hand on your abdomen above the navel and the other hand below the navel. (Fig. 20.12) At the same time gently pump in and up to the cisterna chyli (above angle of right rib cage). Draining the abdomen is important for any health problem below the navel, i.e., digestive problems, hernias in abdominal wall, prostate problems, gynecological problems, hemorrhoids or low back or sciatic pain.

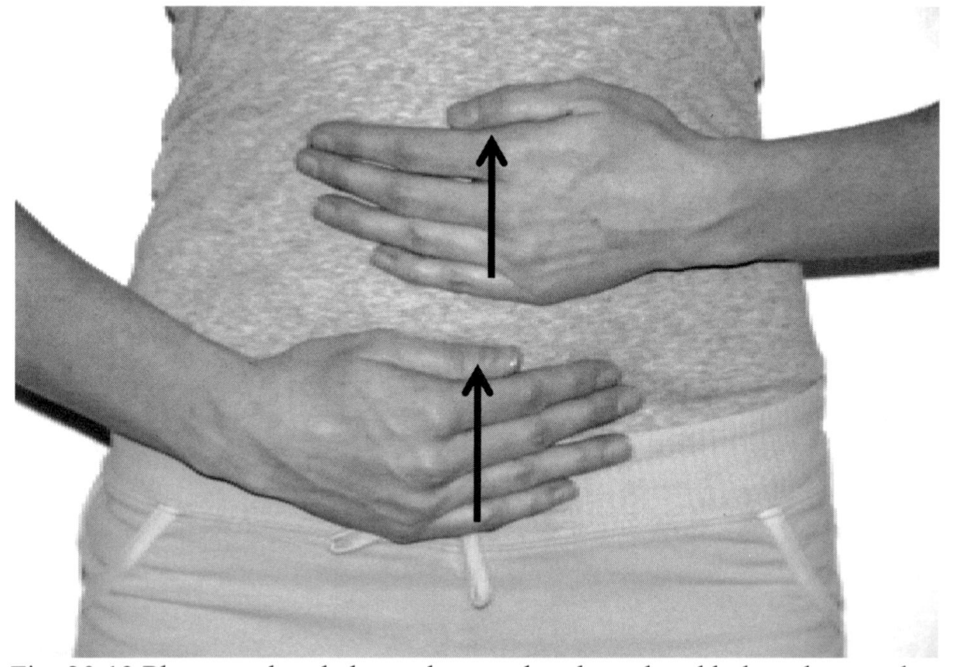

Fig. 20.12 Place one hand above the navel and one hand below the navel.

12. Inguinal Nodes

The inguinal nodes are in the crease at the top of the leg. (Fig. 20.13) When draining the inguinal nodes include the soft area just below the crease, this area also has many lymph nodes. You can effectively drain your inguinal area while laying flat on your back, sitting or standing.

Place the heel of your hand gently onto the tissue just beneath the crease of the leg. Gently pump in and up into the crease and surrounding tissue with a rhythmic wave-like motion. Your focus should be on the heel of the hand but include the whole hand into this gentle motion, in order to drain more of the nodes and surrounding tissue.

Most of the time the lymph system doesn't need much coaxing to begin flowing. When your inguinal nodes are congested, you may have a lack of circulation in your legs or feet, heel spurs, foot pain, sensitive feet, itchy legs, toenail fungus, neuroma's, gout, swelling, cellulite, varicose veins, spider veins, sore knees, hip pain or sciatic pain.

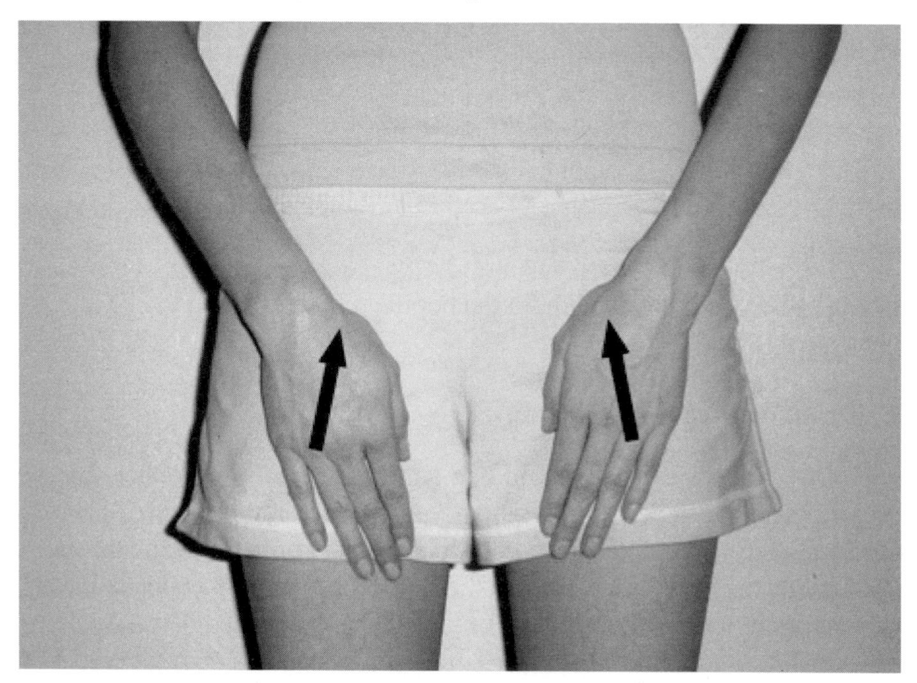

Fig. 20.13 Use the heel and flat part of your hand to gently pump the inguinal nodes, just below the crease of the leg, in and up.

13. Nodes Behind the Knee

Drain the popliteal nodes behind the knee and above the calf to help the deeper lymph flow of the leg (Fig. 20.14). Place your hands behind the knee. Your right hand is on the indentation above the crease and your left hand is on the top portion of the calf just below the knee crease. Your hand position is similar to a grip on a golf club. Pump with the fingers of both hands up the back of leg.

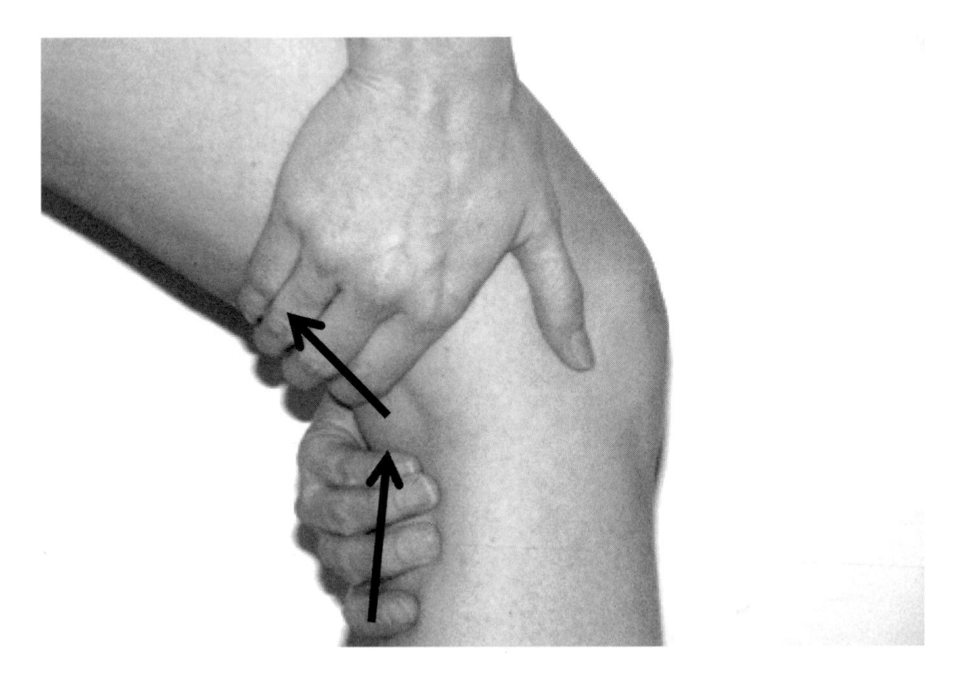

Fig. 20.14 Use both hands to drain the popliteal nodes behind the knee.

14. Drain the Leg

Reach as far down the leg as you can and place a hand on either side (Fig. 20.15). If you can reach your toes put your hands on either side of the foot. Start by sliding your hands down your foot around your ankles and up your leg to just below the knee. This is where the lymph flow from the outside lower leg flows across to join the lymph flow of the inside of the leg.

As you slide your hands up your lower leg, just below the knee, slide your outside hand across to the inside of the leg. Continue bringing both hands up the inside of the leg to just past the knee where both hands fan out to sweep the inside, top and outside of the leg to the inguinal nodes in the crease of the leg. If you have any foot, ankle or leg problems drain the leg and pathway to the main drain often.

If you have a deep vein thrombosis (this is a blood clot in a deeper larger vein of the leg) or have a problem with blood clots, do not drain your legs without first consulting with your health care practitioner.

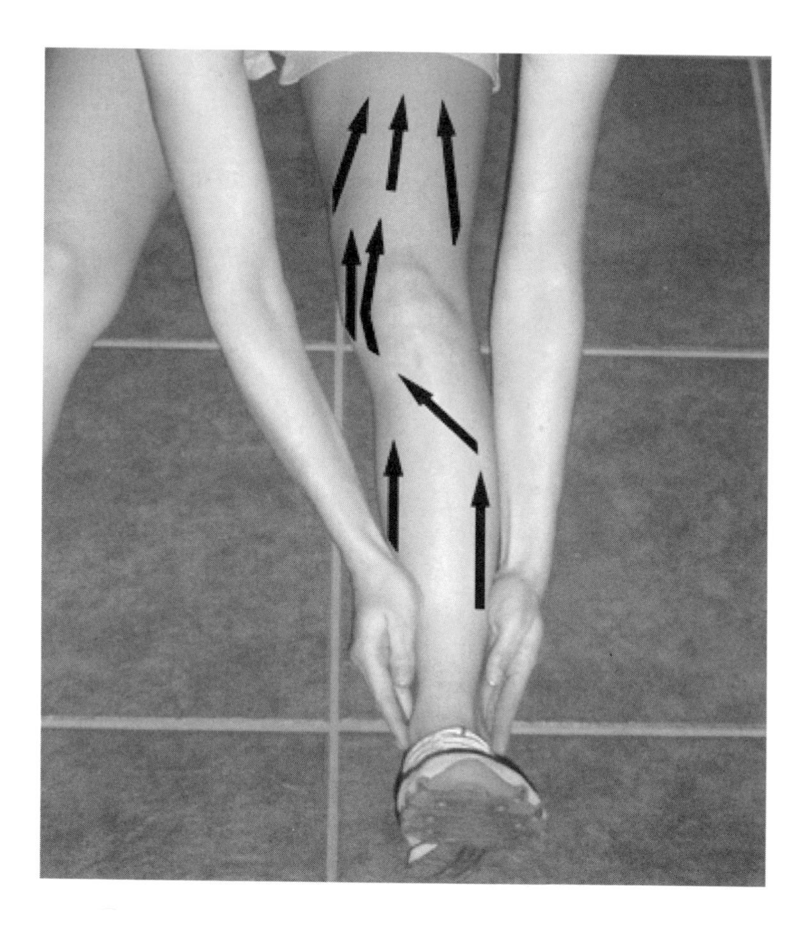

Fig. 20.15 Drain your leg by reaching down as far as you can, pull your hands up in a sweeping motion, up to the inside of the knee and then to the inguinal nodes

When Your in a Rush - Drain the Mother Nodes

The Mother nodes are nodes at the end of an extremity close to the body. When in a rush open the Mother nodes. First, always open the main drain by the clavicles, then open the mother nodes, which are the axilla nodes (underarm) and inguinal nodes (crease at the top of the leg). (Fig. 20.16) When you actively pump these main areas of lymph nodes, as in walking, exercising, bending, reaching or self-lymphatic activation, you are enhancing lymph flow and overall circulation through the tissues. For the arms or legs to drain efficiently the mother nodes of the affected limb need to be pumped to enhance lymph flow out of the extremities.

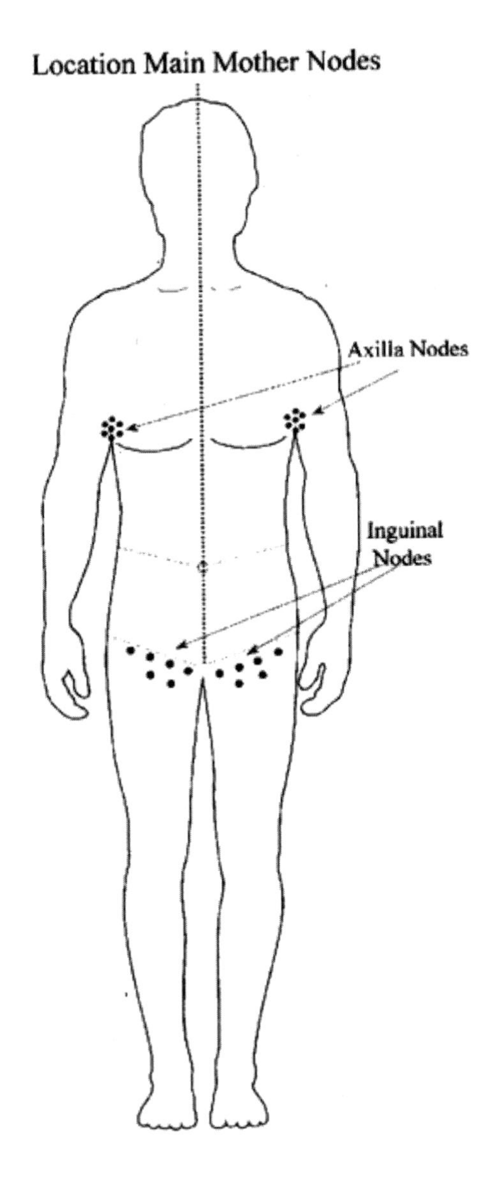

Fig. 20.16 Clusters of lymph nodes in the underarm and in and below the crease of the leg are called Mother Nodes.

Self-Activate Your Lymphatic System

By self-activating your major lymph nodes on a daily basis you can help increase your circulation and reduce your toxicity. Learn to self-activate your lymphatic system using "The Two-Minute Lymph Activation Routine" to increase circulation allowing fresh blood with oxygen and nutrients into the tissue. Enhancing lymph flow increases circulation which allows waste and toxins to leave the tissues. In the Iraq War many soldiers and newspaper personnel sat in vehicles for hours without moving. Many had problems associated with blood clotting and some even died as a result of clots that moved to their heart. A blood clot is a clump of fibrin and other waste that is attached to tissues. If it were to become free and move in your blood stream, it could become a serious life-threatening problem. This simple two-minute routine can be done anywhere, to help move lymph and blood circulation through the tissues to avoid having dangerous blood clots and to improve your health.

In this self-lymphatic activation routine you should drain the nodes gently, pumping them between FIVE to TEN times. When you sweep the skin to the main nodes also sweep lightly between FIVE to TEN times. Start slowly to avoid a healing crisis. This is very gentle work which should never cause pain. Besides your hands you can use a loofah sponge, a dry soft paintbrush (made with a natural bristle) even a small diameter paint roller. While self-activating your lymph take a few sets of two deep breaths, separated by a couple of relaxed breaths to help propel lymph.

The Two-Minute Lymph Activation Routine

Start by taking a few deep breathes, then do a few shoulder shuffles. Alternate your shoulders up and down a few times, don't be afraid to really move them. Moving and stretching your shoulders and neck a few times helps to open the main lymphatic drain. If you have any health concerns check with your health care practitioner before using self-lymphatic activation techniques. Do each of the following techniques five to ten times, start out slowly by doing it every few days. After a week or two you can do the 2-Minute Routine more often until you build up to where you are doing it once or twice a day.

1. Pump Nodes Above Main Drain Down Towards Heart

Gently pump the nodes above the clavicle, in the soft triangle, down to the main drain aiming towards the center of your chest. (Fig. 20.02) Do the right and left side simultaneously or separately, whichever is easier. Your arms can be crossed or uncrossed.

2. Stretch Skin of Neck Down

Drain the skin of your neck down to the clavicle nodes. (Fig. 20.03) Grasp your neck as if you were choking yourself, relax your hands and let them drop so your little fingers are almost touching the clavicle. Flatten your fingers and gently stretch the skin down, aiming under the clavicle bone and release.

3. Stretch Skin at Base of Ear Down

Drain the water wheel (base of the ear) down to the clavicle nodes, do right and left sides at the same time. (Fig. 20.04) Place three fingers to the base of the ear with the middle finger in the crease where the jaw and neck meet. Gently stretch the skin down and release.

4. Sweep Beneath Jaw from Middle of Chin to Ear

Drain the right and left submandibular nodes (beneath the jaw) (Fig. 20.05). Make a soft fist and use your bent fingers to sweep the soft tissue behind the jaw to the ear. Start by the center of your chin and gently sweep to the base of the ear.

5. Sweep from Eyebrows Down to Jaw Line

Drain the inside of the cone of the face down to the nodes below the jaw. (Fig. 20.06) Place your middle fingers along your nose almost touching between your eyebrows. Gently sweep the middle fingers down the side of the nose. As the fingers pass the bridge of the nose, allow your ring, index and little fingers to make contact with the skin and slide down to the jaw line.

6. Pump and Stretch Parotid Nodes to Base of Ear

Drain the parotid nodes (on angle of jaw) to the water wheel (base of the ear) (Fig. 20.07). Place your flat fingers over the angle of the jaw. Your index fingers should be by the by the base of the ear. Gently pump and stretch the skin with your flat fingers, aiming towards the base of the ear.

7. Sweep Forehead to Parotid Nodes

Sweep the forehead and temples down to the parotid nodes (Fig. 20.08). Place the flat part of your fingers to the center of your forehead (fingers tips up) and sweep down over the forehead and temples to the parotid nodes (at the angle of the jaw).

8. Pump Underarm Nodes Towards Heart

Pump, not squeeze, the axilla (underarm) separately, up and into the center of the body towards the heart (Fig. 20.09).

9. Sweep Up Arm into Underarm

Raise your left arm out in front of you, slightly above your heart, with palm facing down. (Fig. 20.10) Place the fingers of your right hand up to the fingers of the left hand. With no added pressure slowly sweep your right hand fingers up the inside (soft part) of the arm into the underarm. Be sure to start your sweep from the tips of your fingers and end deeply in the underarm. Repeat with right arm and hand.

10. Pump Cisterna Chyli Up Along the Right Rib Cage

Pump the cisterna chyli (by angle of right rib cage) up to enhance lymph flow in the abdomen, pelvis and legs (Fig. 20.11). Drain the cisterna chyli by placing your left hand under your right rib cage, the heel of your hand is on the center of your abdomen, your index finger follows the angle of the ribs and your thumb is on top of the ribs. Then place your right hand over your left hand and rhythmically pump with both hands in and down 3-5 times, then up towards the center of your chest 5-10 times. Aim your pumps up towards the heart.

11. Pump Abdomen Above and Below Navel Up

To drain the abdomen place one hand on abdomen above the navel and the other hand below the navel. (Fig. 20.12) At the same time gently pump in and up to the cisterna chyli (angle of right rib cage). Try to create a slow rhythmic wave up to the heart.

12. Pump the Nodes in the Crease of Your Leg Up

Drain the inguinal nodes (in and below the crease of the leg) up towards the heart. (Fig. 20.13) Place the heel of your hand gently onto the tissue just beneath the crease of the leg. Gently pump up into the crease with a rhythmic wave-like motion, include your whole hand to access more lymph nodes and tissue.

13. Pump Nodes Above and Below Back of Knee Up

Drain the nodes behind the knee and calf to help the deeper lymph flow of the leg. (20.14). Place your hands behind the knee. Your right hand is on the indentation above the crease and your left hand is on the top portion of the calf just below the knee crease. Your hand position is similar to a grip on a golf club. Pump with the fingers of both hands up the back of leg.

14. Sweep Up Leg to Inguinal Nodes

While sitting on the floor or in a chair reach as far down the leg as you can and place a hand on either side. (Fig. 20.15) If you can reach your toes, put your hands on either side of the foot. Slide your hands down your foot around your ankles and up your leg to just below the knee. This is where the lymph flow from the outside lower leg flows across to join the lymph flow of the inside of the leg. As you slide your hands up your lower leg, just below the knee, slide your outside hand across to the inside of the leg. Continue bringing both hands up the inside of the leg to just past the knee where both hands fan out to sweep the inside, top and outside of the leg to the inguinal nodes in and below the crease of the leg.

Open the River Before Opening Congested Areas

I often see people rubbing or pressing on an area that might be itchy, tight or sore. In addition to scratching or pressing on the problem area they should open the mother nodes and tissue before the congested area, increasing circulation to the problem. If you have a sore elbow you need to open the nodes above the clavicle and then the underarm nodes to increase lymph flow from the elbow to the main lymph drain. If you have problems or swelling in your legs you should open the nodes above the clavicles. Then open the cisterna chyli, abdominal nodes, inguinal nodes and popliteal nodes. Think of the lymph flow as a river that empties into a vein before the heart. It's important to open the river of lymph starting at the main lymph drain (under left clavicle), then work your way to the problem area. Improve circulation further by then working your way back to the main lymph drain.

Five Steps for Colic, Relaxation and a Happier Baby

Massage and other manual therapies activate the lymph flow and are beneficial for everyone, especially newborn babies and infants. The following five steps are techniques that parents can do to their babies or children once a day. Massaging after a warm bath or at bed time is great, but not right after a feeding. If your child has any health concerns check with your health care practitioner before you try any manual bodywork like massage or lymphatic activation.

1. **Open the main lymphatic drain and the mother nodes**. Stand in front of or sit behind the baby gently place two fingers on each shoulder. Softly pump the baby's left shoulder down towards the feet, then the right shoulder down. Alternate the gentle pumping of the right and left shoulders for a few repetitions. Never force any part of the body.

Activate the lymph in the Mother Nodes 5 times. Start by holding out an arm to the side and gently pump into the underarm towards the heart. Repeat on other side. Move to top of legs beneath crease and gently pump up into crease

2. Open the Cisterna Chyli to aid in relieving abdominal discomfort, chubby legs and for general health. Place your hand or fingers gently on the abdomen, pump slightly in and down to the pelvis 3-5 times, then pump slightly in and up towards the heart 5-10 times. The pump should be slow and very gentle.

3. Massage the baby's muscles with a gentle kneading. You won't need oil or lotion for this type of massage. Place the baby's arm or leg into the palm of your hand. Gently knead the muscle between your thumb and fingers, as if you were kneading special and delicate dough. Start close to the mother nodes (nodes in the underarm or crease of the leg), work your way down the end of the extremity and work your way back to the mother nodes.

4. Gently stretch the baby's arms and legs to increase circulation. Always support the baby's limbs carefully and gently. You can slowly stretch both arms by holding wrist and arm out to the side, then overhead and finish straight out in front. To stretch the legs and low back, gently hold the baby's ankles and lower legs and gently stretch the legs, never force them to straighten. After stretching the baby's legs bend and gently push them into the baby's abdomen a few times; this helps to stretch the low back. Never force any movements. It may take a few stretches or even days or weeks of gentle stretching to coax a limb to relax and fully straighten.

5. While holding the baby in your arms, place one hand very gently on the baby's chest, thumb on one clavicle, 2 or 3 fingers on top of the other clavicle, for five to fifteen minutes. (Fig. 20.17) Your hand should barely rest on the baby's chest, be light enough to allow the baby's chest to move with each breath. If the child is very small, your hand will also be over the abdomen. This is a powerful CranioSacral Therapy technique called the thoracic inlet release. It has the ability to enhance lymph flow and blood circulation in the entire body and head. The main drain of the lymph is by the left clavicle. Placing your fingers on the clavicles opens the main lymph drain and allows for enhanced circulation in the body and head. This technique is "Very Relaxing." It is great to use when a baby or child has colic, earaches, a slight fever, is unable to sleep or is not feeling well. You can use this technique on older children and adults, too. Use a bed or couch or sit in a chair next to the individual to be treated. (Fig. 20.18) The only difference in position is place one hand behind the shoulders and neck for support. Your hand will hold the bump where the neck and shoulders meet.

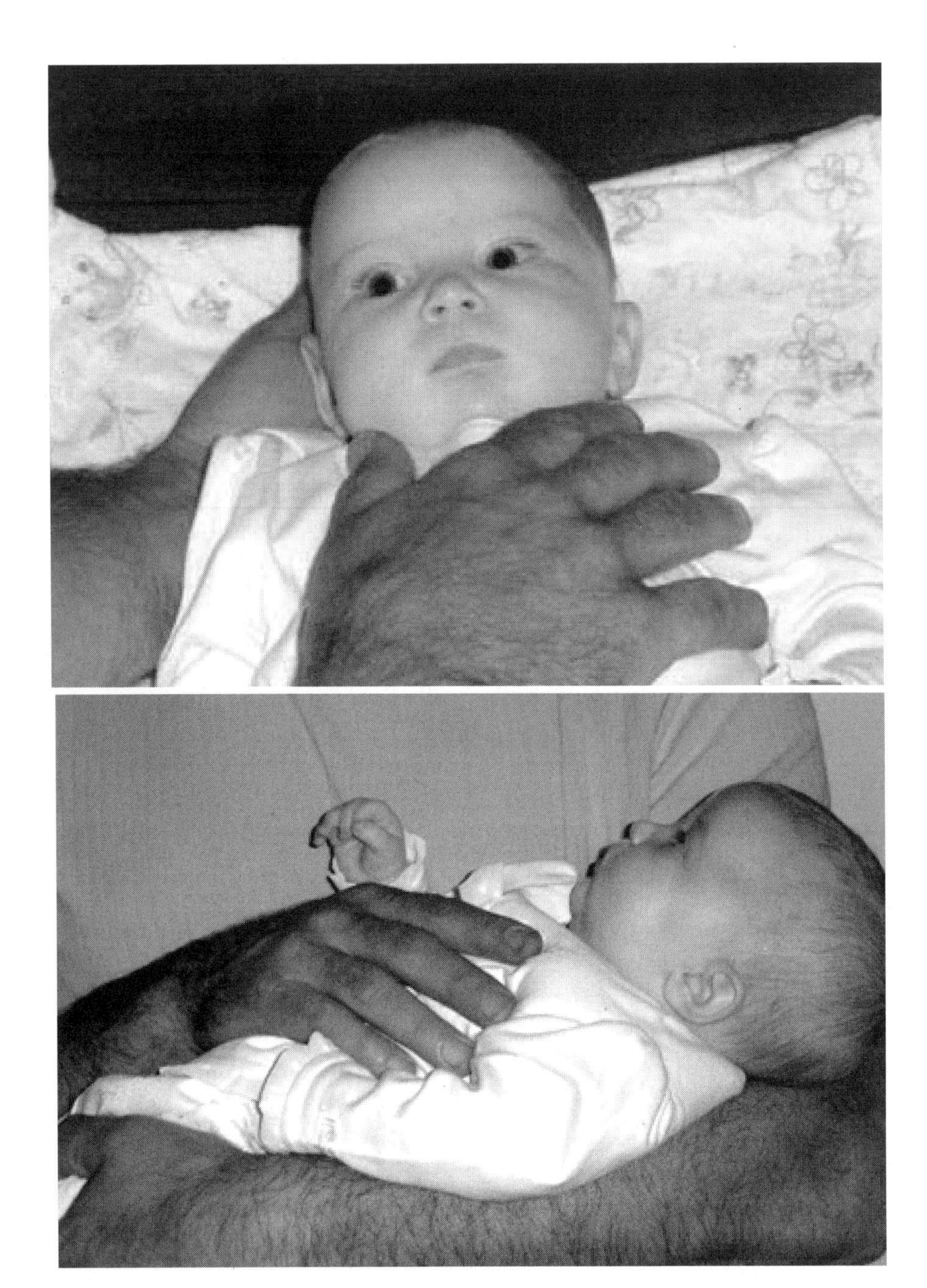

Fig. 20.17 Two easy ways to help relax your children, while increasing their circulation and immune system health. Support the child under the back of the neck and head. Use your other hand to barely make contact with the skin on top of the clavicles.

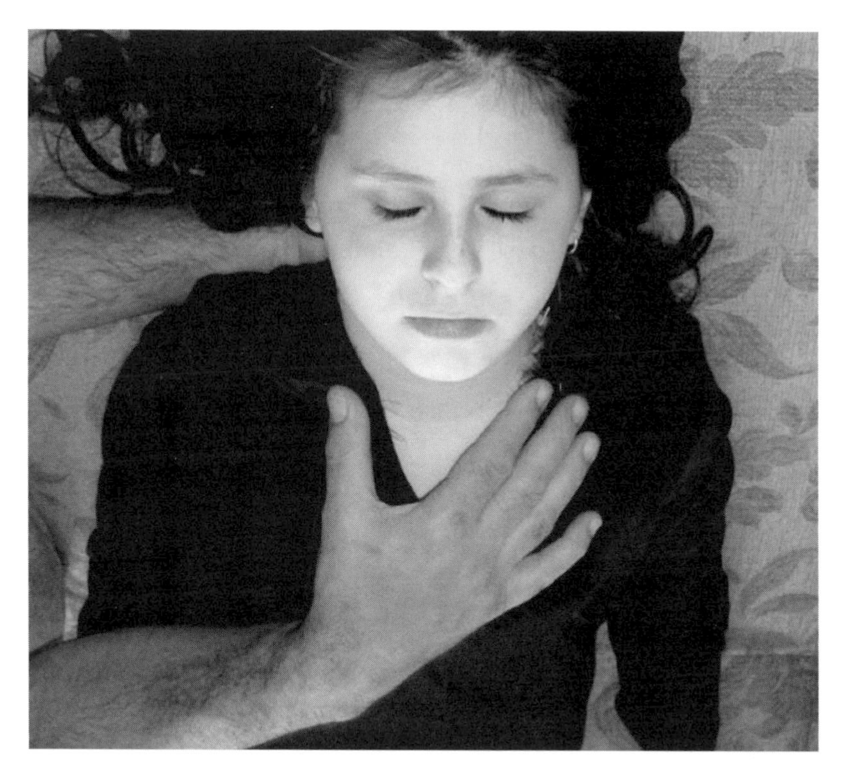

Fig. 20.18 Place one hand behind the shoulders and neck for support and place your other hand on their upper chest with your thumb on one clavicle and your fingers on the other clavicle. Rest the rest of the hand gently on the chest.

Keep Your Lymph Flow Moving

Try this self-help technique next time you are going to lie down. Fill a sandwich size zip lock bag with a half a cup of rice or other grain in it, place in a sock and fold the sock in half and place it on your clavicle bones. You can also use a TV remote control, keys down against your body, on your clavicle bones. After a few minutes you will feel more relaxed. Light pressure on the clavicle bones helps to open the main lymph drain and increases lymph flow and blood circulation in the body and head. Great for sinus problems and relaxtion.

There is no questioning the lymphatic system's important role in maintaining your skin, muscles, tissues, organs, and central nervous system. If you learn to use this emerging science to balance your body to encourage lymph flow and blood circulation you can change your and your family's future. Most importantly you will have a healthier, happier life.

CHAPTER TWENTY-ONE

Responsibility

No One was Interested in the Problem

In trying to get the government's attention to this serious national and world-wide problem, I couldn't believe the enormous amount of run around I experienced. Even the foundations that raise millions of dollars to conquer many diseases such as autism, cancer and MD, had no idea who to refer me to when I called or sent letters asking for help. I knew I had found an important missing key in understanding these diseases and no one was interested.

Should it really have been so difficult to contact someone to alert them to a serious Undetected National Health Problem? Each person I spoke with asked the same question, "What disease are you trying to find out about?" When I would mention that I am trying to alert the government or organization to a possible undetected national health problem, they had no idea where to refer me. Almost everyone I spoke with felt badly that I was getting the run around but they couldn't help.

I called the Mayor of my city to follow up on a letter I had sent asking for help in testing this possible problem. An aide to the mayor sternly said, "The mayor only deals with policies on health, the mayor does not deal with the actual health of its public." This didn't sound right to me. For some reason, people are afraid of this information. What you don't know can seem intimidating and can scare you. In this case what you don't know is killing you.

Individual Responsibility: It is your responsibility to learn this missed information on tissue acidosis and the lymphatic system. Know that there is a problem. You and your family are most probably overly acidic and toxic. Don't panic, check your urine and saliva pH and understand their results. Put the five steps inside this book to rebalance your body and activate your lymphatic system into action for two weeks to a month. You have nothing to lose but your health problems and some weight. Take responsibility for your health. Eat a greener 80/20 diet, fill in with nutritional supplements, begin exercising daily, take two deep breaths often, good posture, drink mineralized water, manage your stress, and have regular sessions of lymphatic activation or self-lymphatic activation. Begin balancing your life today for a healthier and happier tomorrow.

Parental Responsibility: Children learn from watching and imitating their parents. You're not expected to be perfect but you should be setting a good example. You are responsible for your children from conception to when they leave your home. Hopefully in that time they will learn a few healthy habits from you to help them through life. Start teaching your children about balancing their health and self-activating their lymph as soon as they can understand. You will empower them for life by giving them the right information to make the right choices. Know that when you give your children candies, soda and excess acidic foods as more than a rare treat, you are giving them foods that can slow their circulation, make them toxic, hyperactive, or affect their ability to think clearly. Don't blame your child for hyperactive or bad behavior. Up to this point you have been feeding your children; now nourish them and watch them flourish.

National Responsibility: We all need to start taking responsibility. If the basic information in this book makes sense to you, send a letter or e-mail to your mayor, governor, congressmen, senators, and the President. Let them know in writing that you expect immediate government action in dealing with this National Undetected Imbalance. This action should start with the government educating the general public about this simple imbalance, the lymphatic system and how to use this emerging science to prevent disease and improve health.

President, Senators, Congressmen and Elected Politicians' Responsibility: I sincerely love our country. "America, the land of the free!" As Americans we support our President and elected officials; they don't have an easy job. That doesn't mean we like the tremendous amount of pandering between large corporations, drug companies, the FDA and our government. The government is there to protect "The People" not the corporations. Unfortunately, the influence of thousands of corporate lobbyists blinds the politicians. Money can be a very powerful persuader, so your health becomes secondary. You need to take immediate action. Your constituents and immediate family are being hurt from an undetected imbalance that you now know about. Your efforts in dealing with this national problem can either create a healthier future for this great nation or leave our nation with continued declining health and a growing health care crisis. This will become a very large issue in your next election. Your constituency will look to see if you take action to be an advocate for their health or continue to turn your back in favor of corporations. You choose your fate.

Surgeon General's Responsibility: The following duties of The Surgeon General are from their website: "To protect and advance the health of the Nation through educating the public; advocating for effective disease prevention and health promotion programs and activities; and, provide a highly recognized symbol of national commitment to protecting and improving the public's health."

I had the opportunity to speak with the same advisor from the Surgeon General's Office on at least three or four different occasions. We spoke of the letters and research I had sent to advise the Surgeon General's office that there is an undetected tissue acidosis in our nation that needs to be researched further. I could tell I wasn't being taken seriously and that I was becoming an annoyance. I didn't see the focus on "advocating effective disease prevention..." If I had a drug that could solve the problem of tissue acidosis, the advisor may have known where to direct me.

I tried to advise the Surgeon General's office numerous times of an undetected national health problem and no one understood or cared enough to look into this matter further. This is a big problem! Simply educating the public about acid-alkaline balance and the lymphatic system can stem the epidemic of autism, reduce obesity and save the minds of seniors.

Doctor's Responsibility: You have taken a Hippocratic Oath, "first do no harm." Many drugs are harming us. You need to start looking at a new paradigm including acid-alkaline balance, tissue acidosis and a malfunctioning lymphatic system's effect on the body and mind. This is where disease starts.

Our medical system pursues the reduction in symptoms of disease by using medications. As I mentioned before we do need medications in times of trauma, severe disease and in life or death situations. Most of us don't need to be on a drug for a lifetime or for every minor health problem we have, especially when simple lifestyle changes can achieve better results. Educate and empower your patients instead of medicating them.

You need to curb the epidemic levels of childhood diseases, especially autism. This can be achieved by alerting obstetricians that pregnant mothers may be seriously acidic and toxic. Educating mother's and obstetricians about saliva and urine pH testing is the key to stopping infants from having incapacitating diseases. Our children are our future and their future is in your hands.

Medical Insurance Providers' Responsibility: Start a new prevention trend in health care. Start paying and caring for your subscriber's preventative health needs. By preventing disease through regular stress reduction and increased circulation, you may avoid the expensive medications, surgeries and hospital stays. Massage and other science based manual therapies such as CranioSacral Therapy, Lymph Drainage Therapy and Lymphatic Cellular Detox Massage should be covered by insurance.

Corporate Responsibility: The food industry needs an overhaul. Many of our ways to process, store or can food have been utilized for decades. There must be better ways to store or process food to keep all of its flavor and nutritional content intact without adding ascorbic acid which is acid forming. How do we grow food with high levels of nutrients and no chemical pesticides? How do we ensure all produce and livestock coming into this country are free of toxins, bacteria, hormones and food additives? If you produce a very popular food item that is acid producing research and produce a healthier, more alkaline producing version. Many companies are already doing this; those that are not looking to the future will be left behind. Don't replace your product, but have a healthier more alkaline choice for those that are looking for alternatives.

We eat a large amount of pizza in this country. There are over 61,000 pizzerias in the United States. Some of the major pizza chains feed many in our nation on a regular basis. Pizza needs an upgrade. The dough needs to be made healthier by adding whole grains (for example semolina, sprouted wheat, flax meal and whole-wheat flour). Follow Barilla Pasta who made a choice to make a more nutritious pasta by adding healthy grains and legumes. Use quality oil, such as olive oil, instead of hydrogenated oils in making dough. The tomato sauce needs to be fresher and made more alkaline and the cheese should be a whole milk product applied lightly to the pizza. Original pizza makers that came from Italy to this country added very little cheese. Our pizzas today are laden with processed white flour, hydrogenated oils, pepperoni and too much processed cheese. They need to, and can be, made healthier. Even burgers and chicken sandwiches can be made healthier by adding whole-wheat buns, extra lettuce, tomato, onion and avocado. A healthier burger can be made with ground turkey instead of beef. As awareness of Acid-Alkaline Balance grows consumers will be looking for healthier alternatives to high acid foods.

Balancing the World

If the steps in this book, particularly the "80/20 Diet", were followed nationally, the world, as we now know it, would actually change, becoming more in balance. Farmers would be able to make a living with the increased demand for produce. Our demand for meats and poultry would be reduced, cutting down on the amount of animal waste that is currently a toxic problem polluting surrounding soil and water supplies. Eating less fish would bring our oceans and streams back into balance by reducing over fishing. Help yourself, your family and help bring the world back into balance; eat more vegetables, fruit and some whole grains.

5 Steps to Balance, Lymph Activation and Optimal Health

1. **Learn Your Warning Signs Of Toxicity.** Find out if you are "Out of Balance" and learn your warning signs of toxicity in your body.

2. **Green-Up Your Diet "80/20 Rule."** Eat an 80% Alkaline and 20% Acid Diet. Learn the benefits of taking nutritional supplements, alkalizing products and systemic enzymes.

3. **Increase Your Circulation:** Exercise, Deep Breathing, Hydration and Posture

4. **Stress Reduction:** Receive a massage and try daily meditation to relax and increase your blood flow.

5. **Manual Detoxification – The Real Key to Optimal Health**
   Lymphatic Activation or Self-Lymphatic Activation

A Healthy and Happy Life Begins with Balance

REFERENCES

Information on health, pH and the lymph system is referenced from the following books on pH, medical texts, The Merck Manual and the Internet.

Silent Waves, Theory and Practice of Lymph Drainage Therapy by Bruno Chikly, M.D., DO. (hon)

CranioSacral Therapy by John E. Upledger, D.O., F.A.A.O.

Alkalize or Die by Theodore A. Baroody, N.D.

Sick and Tired? by Robert O. Young, Ph.D,, Shelley Redford Young, L.M.T.

The pH Miracle by Robert O. Young, Ph.D,, Shelley Redford Young, L.M.T.

The Acid-Alkaline Balance Diet by Felicia Drury Kliment

The Master Cleanser by Stanley Burroughs

The Body's Many Cries For Water by F. Batmanghelidj, M.D.

Atlas of Human Anatomy by Frank H. Netter, M.D.

The Merck Manual, Seventeenth Edition

Search the Internet

Acidosis, acid–alkaline balance, acidic pH, low pH, acid imbalance

---

ALS

http://www.ninds.nih.gov/disorders/amyotrophiclateralsclerosis/amyotrophiclateralsclerosis.htm#What_is

Alzheimer's Tau Protein

http://www.therubins.com/alzheim/alzbrain21.htm

Amyloidosis

http://www.mayoclinic.com/health/amyloidosis/DS00431

Artheriosclerosis

http://www.nlm.nih.gov/medlineplus/ency/article/000171.htm

Autism

http://en.wikipedia.org/wiki/Autism

Batten Disease
http://en.wikipedia.org/wiki/Batten_disease
Brain Swelling
http://hosting.texoma.net/business/biotech/thia-faq.htm
C-Reactive Protein
http://www.americanheart.org/presenter.jhtml?identifier=4648
Chemical Sensitivity
http://www.merck.com/mmhe/sec25/ch306/ch306d.html
Chronic Fatigue Syndrome
http://en.wikipedia.org/wiki/Chronic_fatigue_syndrome
Cow's Milk Not for Babies
http://www.nlm.nih.gov/medlineplus/ency/article/002448.htm
CSF Fetus
http://nro.sagepub.com/cgi/content/short/6/2/77
CSF Lymph Connection
http://ajpregu.physiology.org/cgi/content/abstract/272/5/R1613
Depleted Uranium
http://archives.cnn.com/2000/WORLD/europe/09/03/france.gulf/
Diabetes Studies
http://diabetes.diabetesjournals.org/cgi/content/abstract/30/5/402
http://diabetes.diabetesjournals.org/cgi/content/abstract/34/8/744
Enzyme Production
http://www.totalityofbeing.com/EFMain.htm
Fibromyalgia
http://fmaware.org/fminfo/brochure.htm#symptoms
Food Pyramid
http://www.cbsnews.com/stories/2004/11/21/sunday/main656834.shtml
Gulf War Syndrome
http://en.wikipedia.org/wiki/Gulf_War_syndrome
Heart Circulation, aneurysm, and edema
http://www.accessexcellence.org/AE/AEC/CC/heart_anatomy.html
Heart Vasospasm
http://encarta.msn.com/vasospasm.html
High Blood Pressure
http://en.wikipedia.org/wiki/Hypertension
Hippocrates
http://massagetherapy.suite101.com/article.cfm/hippocrates_and_massage
http://www.whoosh.org/issue30/bremer6.html#backnote02

Hypo-Hyperthyroid
http://www.swedish.org/17344.cfm
Kidney
http://coe.fgcu.edu/faculty/greenep/kidney/Glomerulus.html
Lance Armstrong
http://www.cyclingnews.com/results/archives/oct96/lance.html
Leukemia
http://www.mdanderson.org/departments/leukemia/dIndes.cfm?pn=A8426C6A-D0FF-11D4-80FD00508B603A14
Lymph Makes Us Fat
http://www.ncbi.nlm.nih.gov/entrez/query.fcgi?cmd=Retrieve&db=PubMed&list_uids=16170315&dopt=Citation
Lymphatic Vascular Defects Cause Adult-Onset Obesity
http://www.nature.com/ng/journal/v37/n10/abs/ng1005-1023.html
Mad Cow
http://www.cnn.com/2003/US/12/23/mad.cowhttp://www.drday.com/madcow.htm
Max Heart Rate Chart
http://www.americanheart.org/presenter.jhtml?identifier=4736
Meditation
http://www.scienceblog.com/cms/node/7121
Meningitis
http://en.wikipedia.org/wiki/Meningitis
Muscular Dystrophy
http://www.healthscout.com/ency/68/451/main.html#DefinitinofMuscularDystrophy
Multiple Sclerosis
http://www.ninds.nih.gov/disorders/multiple_sclerosis/multiple_sclerosis.htm
Nephritis / Childhood Hypertension
http://www.emedicine.com/ped/topic1561.htm
Pancreatic Proteolytic Enzymes
http://www.ncbi.nlm.nih.gov/entrez/query.fcgi?cmd=Retrieve&db=PubMed&list_uids=10368805&dopt=Citation
Pizza Statistics
http://pizzaware.com/facts.htm
Protein in Foods
http://www.annecollins.com/protein-foods.htm
Protein Needs
http://www.annecollins.com/protein-needs-diet.htm

Removing poisons
http://www.massagemag.com/Magazine/2005/issue113/history113.php
Rocket Fuel Chemicals Found in Breast Milk
http://www.livescience.com/health/050224_rocket_fuel.html
Straterra Black Box Warning
http://www.fda.gov/CDER/DRUG/advisory/atomoxetine.htm
Teen Suicide
http://www.aacap.org/publications/factsfam/suicide.htm
Warfarin and Vitamin K
http://arbl.cvmbs.colostate.edu/hbooks/pathphys/misc_topics/vitamink.html
Water Cure
http://www.watercure.com/products/books.html
Wheat Germ
http://www.wisegeek.com/what-is-wheat-germ.htm
Viagra
http://www.cbsnews.com/stories/2004/11/15/health/main655894.shtml
Viagra Vision Problems
http://www.cnn.com/2005/HEALTH/conditions/05/29/viagra.gupta/

RESOURCES

Lymphatic Wellness Center
Lymphatic Activation
Wickenburg, Arizona
1-928-684-8946
www.HealthyLymphSystem.com

LL's Magnetic Clay
Detox Clay Baths
1-800-257-3315
www.magneticclay.com

Natural Vitality
Peter Gilham's Natural Calm
1-800-446-7462
www.vites.com

Needak Manufacturing
The "Soft Bounce" Rebounder
1-800-232-5762
www.needak-rebounders.com

Organic Frog
Greens Today- Vegan Formula
1-866-403-2247
www.organicfrog.com

pHion Nutrition
pH Test Strips
1-888-744-8589
www.ph-ion.com

Purity Products
Perfect Multi Super Greens
Triple Greens Powder
1-800-256-6102
www.purityproducts.com

SeaAloe Inc.
SeaAloe
1-800-732-1150
www.myseaaloe.com

Vaxa International
Buffer – pH+, pH Test Strips
1-877-622-8292 (VAXA)
www.bufferph.com

WAM Essentials, Inc.
Zymessence
Systemic Enzyme Blend
1-866-268-3216
www.DocsPrefer.com

The Upledger Institute
Find a CranioSacral
or Lymph Drainage Therapist
www.upledger.com

Quick Order Form

Fax Orders: (948) 684-3781

Telephone Orders Monday - Friday: 1-800-214-8110

Online: www.acid-imbalance.com Save Shipping Order Online

Postal Orders: Vision Publishing, LLC
PO Box 2122
Wickenburg, AZ 85358

Please send the following books. I understand that I may return the item if you have not gained from the information within.

____

____

Please send more FREE information on:

☐ Other Books ☐ Speaking/Seminars ☐ Consulting

Name:____

Address:______________________________________

City:________________________ State:____ Zip:__________

Telephone:____________________ email:__________________

Sales tax: Please add 8%

Shipping: $4.00 for first book, $2.00 for each additional copy

International: $9.00 for first book, $5.00 for each additional copy

Payment: ☐ Check ☐ Visa ☐ M/C ☐ Amex ☐ Discover

Card #:______________________________ Exp. date:________

Name on card: ____________________________________

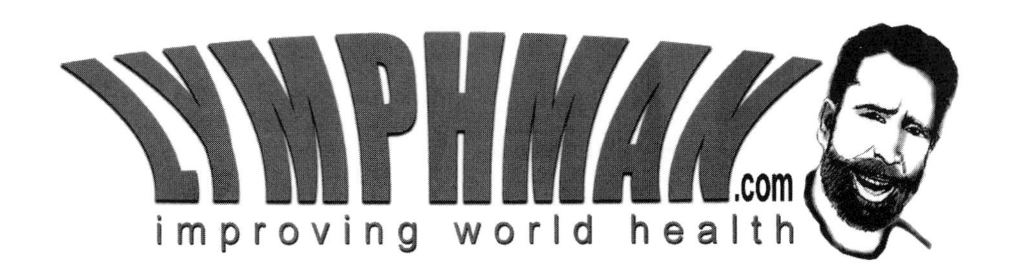

A Simple Imbalance is Probably Hurting You and Your Children

Hi, this is John Ossipinsky, author of *An Undetected Acid-Alkaline Imbalance*. If you have been looking for answers for your fatigue, headaches, migraines, insomnia, cancer, heart disease, swelling, inability to think and depression then you have to visit me at LymphMan.com to become Empowered to create health.

In 2003 I realized that the nation, and probably the world, was suffering from An Undetected Acid-Alkaline Imbalance. This simple imbalance is a serious mattter, acid is hurting most of you, especially children and no one is aware that acid is anything more than a digestive problem.

At LymphMan.com you will benefit from my over fourteen years of studying and working with the lymphatic system. The lymphatic system is an emerging science that you must understand to create health. Within a few days of joining LymphMan.com you will understand the lymphatic systems importance in improving and maintaining your health and mind. You will also know how to self-activate your lymphatic system to improve your circulation and health.

LymphMan.com is the next evolution in my quest to "improve world health." My hope is that LymphMan.com becomes your lymphatic medicine cabinet. A place where you turn to find answers to improve your health naturally. Visit me at www.LymphMan.com and learn the proper care and maintenance of your lymphatic system, for a Healthier, Happier Life. You Deserve It!

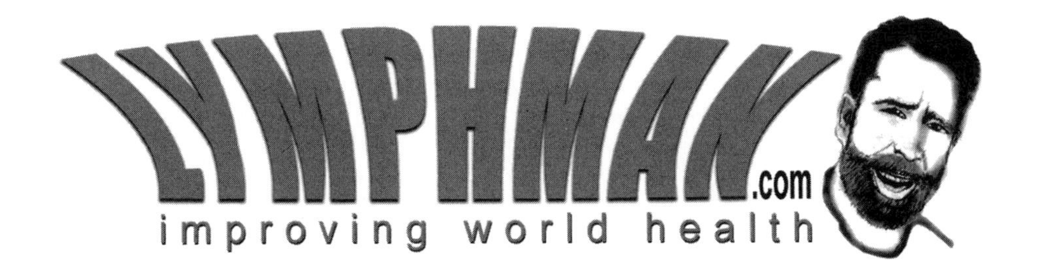

Over Thirty Easy to Follow Videos Explaining:

The Importance of the Lymphatic System
How Acid is Hurting You
5 Steps to Balance, Lymph Activation and Health
Healthy Cooking Demonstrations

Self-Lymphatic Activation to:
Help Aches, Pains and Insomnia
Improve Circulation
Improve Immune System
Improve Ability to Think
Help with Weight Loss
Help Clear Skin
Improve Healing
Slow Aging

Learn How to Easily Activate the Lymphatics in:
Infants and Children
Reduces Colic, Earaches, Irritability, Skin Problems

Bed or Wheelchair Bound Family Members
Improves Circulation, Immune System and Overall Health

Dogs, Cats and Horses
Mammals have a lymphatic system and their health benefits from lymphatic activation